HIGH VIBRATIONAL WELLNESS

INTUITIVE HEALING THERAPIES TO NOURISH YOUR BODY TEMPLE

LAINIE SEVANTE WULKAN

FEATURING: RUTH S. BAILEY, KARI BOZIC, LISA BROWN, TAMMY "TLC" LYNN CALDERON, SUSAN G. CHAMBERLAIN, JOY E. DAVIS, SUSAN WALLACE DONEGAN, JULIANNE FARRELL, JOSEPH M. FASI II, DENISE FLOOD, CAROLYN NICHOLSON FOWLER, DR. CHERYLE FREEDMAN, DR. VITO KOSTRZEWSKI, KANDY TAYLOR LOVE, CAROLINE MARY, LINDA McBEE, HANNAH McKITRICK, ANGELA ORORA MEDWAY-SMITH, DARYL L. MOUNTFORD, JANET NAMASTE, KAREN RUDOLF, T. BRANDON RUSS, NYDIA LAYSA STONE, CHARLOTTE WARN

HIGH VIBRATIONAL WELLNESS

INTUITIVE HEALING THERAPIES
TO NOURISH YOUR BODY TEMPLE

LAINIE SEVANTE WULKAN

FEATURING: RUTH S. BAILEY, KARI BOZIC, LISA BROWN, TAMMY "TLC" LYNN CALDERON, SUSAN G. CHAMBERLAIN, JOY E. DAVIS, SUSAN WALLACE DONEGAN, JULIANNE FARRELL, JOSEPH M. FASI II, DENISE FLOOD, CAROLYN NICHOLSON FOWLER, DR. CHERYLE FREEDMAN, DR. VITO KOSTRZEWSKI, KANDY TAYLOR LOVE, CAROLINE MARY, LINDA McBEE, HANNAH McKITRICK, ANGELA ORORA MEDWAY-SMITH, DARYL L. MOUNTFORD, JANET NAMASTE, KAREN RUDOLF, T. BRANDON RUSS, NYDIA LAYSA STONE, CHARLOTTE WARN

NOURISHING REVIEWS

"You will enjoy *High Vibrational Wellness,* a gem of a book, as much as I did, whether you read a quote, passage, chapter or more. It's a deep remembering, which touches the soul part that's the same in us all. Each of the 25 Authors guides us through a spiritual smorgasbord of experiences, downloads, energies and recoveries, enabling both the advanced and beginners to be escorted and exposed to the secrets of life, beyond the unknown."

~ **Patrick Conlon,** Founder of Enlightened Energetics – A multi-modality healing practice in Cape Coral, Florida and globally online

"*High Vibrational Wellness* is a potent tool for transformation on all levels of your physical, mental, emotional and spiritual well-being. Lainie Sevante Wulkan's passion for and dedication to holistic health is the guiding light for this collaborative creation that will inspire, uplift and enlighten your path!"

~ **Teressena Bakens,** Creatix, Medicine Woman, creator of *The Fifth Tarot: Alchemy of the Five Elements* and Author of *Cosmic Odyssey,* Co-Facilitator of *Joie de Vivre Retreats*

"*High Vibrational Wellness* is fertile with a variety of enlightened perspectives and alternative, healing nourishment. Our world is deeply in need of the wisdom contained and "spelled" out within these pages. This collaboration fills a gap in existing literature, so richly filled with profound energy emitted by the Author's voices and their healing information to make it accessible to each reader."

~ **Keely Mackey-Gonzales,** aka Celloquacious multi-award winning cellist, composer, interdisciplinary artist and educator

"Reading and experiencing the essence of all that has been shared in *High Vibrational Wellness,* I can truly say these stories are my stories and yours: those we've written, are writing and have yet to write. They hold hidden treasures to vibrating in higher and higher frequencies in all ways. Take your time to absorb the wonders of this Divine banquet of wisdom as it will transform you in unimaginable ways."

~ **Timothy Stuetz,** Author of 175+ children's books and Teacher of Meditation, Reiki, T'ai Chi/Qigong and Yoga

"Ready for adventure? Grab onto the railing and sail with the powerful waves of soul stories from the courageous authors of *High Vibrational Wellness*! Watch each author encounter their big wave, and transform themselves, finding their soul-satisfying bliss. Let's face it, we live on planet earth, so having a great set of body-mind-spirit tools available for daily use is essential. These authors answered the call. *High Vibrational Wellness* offers a treasure chest of tools which will help you get off that sand bank you may be stuck on and put your life on its grandest course!"

~ **Deb Martin,** Co-Owner of Lotus Blossom Clinic, Holistic Health Educator and Practitioner

"First, wrap our minds around the fact food has a message for you. Food has a vibration frequency from the plant itself and its color. Lainie Sevante Wulkan has created an information library in one book, loaded with tools and inspiration that will expand your own personal health. I love the thought of "soul shopping"(Chapter 1) and how every day is an opportunity to nourish more than your body."

~ **Sandra McGill,** Multi – Modality Healer and Author of Jesus Healing Codes, My Best Friend Pet Cards and two short angel stories

"I've seen and worked with a lot of healers in the 20+ years I've been producing national spiritual festivals and am incredibly delighted to see this fresh perspective to wellness, particularly a full rounded approach to all the bodies we have - emotional, mental, physical and spiritual. Kudos to Lainie Sevante Wulkan and her inspiring Co-Authors for this triumphant collaboration in *High Vibrational Wellness.*"

~ **Mary Ellen Popyk,** Founder of The Sanctuary for Mind, Body & Spirit and Producer of National Spirit Fest Expos and the Wisdom of Light Conference

"*High Vibrational Wellness* most assuredly could change your life! Each chapter is a rarified sharing and forthright biographical story which profoundly answers wellness questions you may never have thought to ask. Buy this book for friends and family, but most importantly, buy it for YOURSELF!"

~ **Patricia DeGrood,** Global retreat Yoga Instructor, MS in Health Education and Owner of Do You Yoga

DISCLAIMER

This book is designed to provide competent, reliable, and educational information regarding health, wellness, nutritional, and other subject matter covered. However, it is sold with the understanding the authors and publisher specifically disclaim all responsibility for any liability, loss, or risk, personal or otherwise, incurred as a consequence, directly or indirectly, of the use and application of any of the contents of this publication.

In order to maintain the anonymity of others, the names and identifying characteristics of some people, places, and organizations described in this book have been changed.

This publication contains content that may be potentially triggering or disturbing. Individuals who are sensitive to certain themes are advised to exercise caution while reading.

The opinions, ideas, and recommendations contained in this publication do not necessarily represent those of the Publisher. The use of any information provided in this book is solely at your own risk.

Know that the experts here have shared their tools, practices, and knowledge with you with a sincere and generous intent to assist you on your business journey. Please contact them with any questions you may have about the techniques or information they provided. They will be happy to assist you further and be an ongoing resource for your success!

FOREWORD

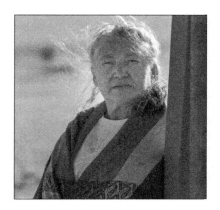

Beloved Friends and Family in the Four Directions:

Blessings to you and the journey that has led you here. I've known Sevante for more than 15 years, and it has always been clear to me that her purpose is to move the world forward in a positive way. Her passion for honoring Mother Earth in all her glory is very aligned with mine, and we've had many opportunities to create works for humanity and the preservation of the planet together.

Years, ago when I recorded the Grandmother's Prayer for Humanity album which raised money for my seed temple at her husband's recording studio, we shared conversations about nature, the elements, the preservation of seeds, healing foods, the Earth, and the vital importance of honoring Creator's blessings given to us from the bushes and trees which provide the sustenance for our bodies and spirit to heal.

I watched her become "The Food Oracle" and bring forward a very unique path of bridging spirit and science together with The Food Healing Oracle Deck® series to a worldwide stage. These truly original decks provide channeled healing wisdom and practical nutritional information to better understand your food choices and allow you to see inherently that there are deeper messages to be gleaned from the Divine. She teaches us through her organization, CIFT (Center for Intuitive Food Therapy™), that we have the answers already inside and that spending time in meditation and prayer further develops our intuition and connection to source, thus allowing us a greater existence to navigate our human experience.

Now, with *High Vibrational Wellness – Intuitive Healing Therapies to Nourish Your Body Temple*, Sevante has brought not only her profound knowledge of Mother Nature's wisdom to the forefront for the reader's consideration, but she also assembled a very dynamic and thoughtful group of global healers who also share a passion for healing in a variety of powerful and essential ways.

As demonstrated so beautifully and artfully, how we feed our body temple is more than just the food we put inside. There is a responsibility we are given as stewards of the Creator to feed our minds and soul with the sacred sacrament of positive thinking and being so we can then be that for others.

The world is at a pivotal time and the importance of taking care of ourselves so we can take care of others has never been more important.

I have gathered my indigenous sisters—fellow grandmothers from the four corners who also share the same concerns as Sevante and myself—to find ways to come to a greater place of enlightenment and peace. This only can begin from inside, and *High Vibrational Wellness* offers many gifts to choose that pathway to learn to resonate at a higher level of self-care so that transformative wisdom can be modeled for others.

I know this book will inspire you to see Mother Nature differently and realize that we're all connected, from being nature ourselves to being in one accord with the five elements and all its inhabitants, including the winged ones and four-leggeds. May you find this book to be an essential guide for making a deeper connection to Source and activating another level of understanding of the greater messages from the cosmos.

May you be truly nourished in your mind, body, and spirit.

With great honor and respect,
Grandmother Flordemayo

Curandera Espiritu, Healer of Divine Spirit

Founder of The Path – <u>GrandmotherFlordemayo.com</u>

Founding Member of The Confederation of Indigenous Elders of the America (1995-2000), Institute of Natural and Traditional Knowledge (2003- 2007) Church of the Spiritual Path (1998, 2008-2014), The International Council of Thirteen Indigenous Grandmothers (2004 -2014)

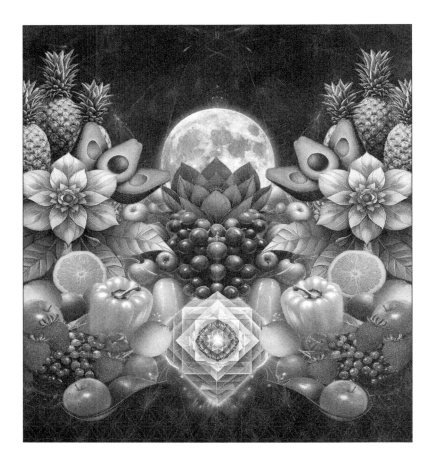

Ramona Teo is a visionary artist and graphic designer from New Mexico. The core theme found throughout most of her work is the mandala, or sacred circle. She works with many artistic mediums including colored pencil, acrylic and digital illustration. The cover art for this book was designed using a combination of AI generated images and Ramona's digital illustration and collage techniques.

Connect with Ramona:

Website: divinenaturearts.com

Facebook: facebook.com/ramona.teo

Instagram: instagram.com/divine.nature.arts

Etsy: divinenaturearts.etsy.com

DEDICATION

I dedicate this book to my family. They're my compass and guiding light.

To my brilliant and loving husband, Howard Merlin Wulkan. You make every day a delicious meal and I am grateful for your continued support, allowing me to nourish my ideas, adventures, and wanderlust.

To my beautiful daughters, Heather and Sarah, I love that you have embraced the importance and reverence for food in your own unique ways. I'm incredibly proud of you both.

To my mom, Mickey. You were the first to teach me at a young age about nutrition and wellness. While at the time I thought your "more than three, leave it be" (referring to ingredients) was outlandish and bizarre, I see now how right you were in opening up my awareness to staying as close to Mother Nature to eat.

Lastly, to my Food Healing Oracle Deck® and CIFT (Center for Intuitive Food Therapy™) "cherries" (community). You have made this journey so wonderful and I am grateful for all of you who have joined this vortex of nourishment to awaken humanity to Spirit's deeper messages in food.

Table of Contents

INTRODUCTION

Welcome to your journey of enlightened healing. I'm truly grateful you're honoring yourself and others by choosing to read *High Vibrational Wellness – Intuitive Healing Therapies to Nourish Your Body Temple.*

This book offers a bounty of wisdom, love, and awareness to bring you back to center, to the essence of your core sense of self.

When one's soul is asking for an upgrade to emotional, mental, physical and/or spiritual wellness, a cleansing path to mind, body and spirit is called into being. We heard your call. This is *the* book to bring your journey to the next level of health, wealth and liberation.

I'm proud to bring you a source of inspiration, care, consideration, and achievement from the 25 expert authors on these pages. These incredibly talented and conscious writers have opened up their hearts and minds to bring you into their personal and professional worlds to share with you their vulnerability, humanity, and journey into transformation. They have dedicated themselves to bettering the world so you can rise as a collective to greater change, starting with yourselves.

At a time on the planet when life is moving at record speed, I'm still surprised by how quickly time flies. Many of you are existing on autopilot, eating with the "grab-n-go" philosophy, exercising less, and becoming more sedentary. You want to make a change and your soul has been giving you the "little knocks" on the door, an awareness that something's got to give. What signs are you experiencing?

Whether there's an increase in aching joints or weight gain, more occurrences of illness, or perhaps mood fluctuations in anxiety and depression, the time to take notice is now. In some cases, a bigger knock you weren't expecting, such as a diagnosis, arrives. Regardless of circumstance, you've come to a safe zone in which you least expected it. These bumps or boulders can provide greater insight into where to go next.

You are ever-evolving, and while you are here on this planet of learning, there is always an opportunity to shift into the next greater version of yourself, the one that is calling you now to wake up, peel the layers of discontent back, and begin to shine brightly.

While many of you are interested in *feeding* your physical body, others are here to learn how to *feed your mind* and/or *Soul*. Food comes in many forms, and your body temple needs all four bodies (emotional, mental, physical, and spiritual) to be in balance so it can support your greatest upliftment. Let the nutrition from these incredible authors nourish your needs.

Are you ready to listen? The lines are open, and we're ready to serve.

Blessings to you on this journey of wellness and the path to greater consciousness in all areas of your life. Here's to making profound and instantaneous shifts. You are here. We are here together. Settle in and enjoy this journey of profound wisdom and healing.

To your infinite nourishment,

Lainie Sevante Wulkan

CHAPTER 1

YOUR COSMIC ROADMAP TO CONSCIOUS EATING

ACTIVATING YOUR INTUITION FOR HIGH VIBRATIONAL WELLNESS

Lainie Sevante Wulkan, Intuitive Food Therapist

MY STORY

"I have heart disease and don't know what to do," said the holistic fair attendee faintly as she lowered her head in defeat. She looked as though her world was falling out from under her. As an empath, I felt her pain.

As she looked around my Food Healing Oracle Deck® booth, I watched her expression alternate between intrigue and curiosity to trepidation and fear. She probably had never spoken to a "Food Oracle" before. Most people haven't. Her mind appeared to be spinning a hundred miles an hour. She was looking for answers and needed them fast.

I've seen that look many times before. Just that day, she was nearly the hundredth person I read for at the holistic fair, where I introduced my new oracle book and card set about Spirit's deeper messages hidden in food.

Angels be with her now. She needs a sign she's on the right road to somewhere.

I said a prayer to the higher realms, asked that the perfect card be drawn for her highest good, fanned them out for her to choose, and watched with great anticipation as she pulled one and turned it over.

Red Bell Peppers - Inspiration.

Bullseye. Perfect card, indeed. Thank you, Spirit.

"Wonderful pick," I shared. "Red bell peppers are excellent for cardiovascular care. National Institute of Health studies show the carotenoid phytochemicals in red bell peppers, their antioxidants and anti-inflammatory effects are superior for heart health. That's why it's our *INSPIRATION* card. Next time you slice into one, notice how they look like the chambers of a heart."

She looked down at the card and then up at me in bewilderment, commenting how she loves red bell peppers and didn't know they were good for her. She smiled and appeared eager to learn more.

Thanks, Mother Nature. This never gets old.

Another time, I visited a friend and offered her a reading. I sensed her adrenals were shot, noticed her cadence was slow, and heard the fatigue in her voice.

"I have adrenal fatigue," she said. *Yep. Knew that one was coming.*

"Pull a card and see what food will be good to eat," I responded. She had not seen The Food Healing Oracle Deck® before and was game for seeing what the cards might reveal.

She picked **Asparagus - Transformation.**

Ding, ding, ding, ding!

"You picked a winner," I said with a Cheshire cat's grin. "To boost your adrenals, you'll want to rid the system of excess toxins and waste. To do that, you need to support the work of the liver, and asparagus is your best friend. Clean up the crud in your system and watch your energy return."

Later that day, a nutritionist with millions of followers posted a blog about adrenal fatigue. His number one recommendation? Yep—

asparagus. I love third-party validation. I sent my friend the link to give her confirmation that her card pull was accurate. She couldn't believe it. But, I could. I've seen it time and time again.

Like the asparagus, she did end up having quite the transformation. She ate asparagus that week, upped her water intake, backed off sugars, and began to feel better emotionally, mentally, physically, and even spiritually.

Get the teachings out there. There's more to our dinner plate than meets the eye. The world must know that important messages are right under our noses for health and longevity.

Self-talk is essential for me to keep on track. "Food Talk" is brave, new territory to show people through an oracle deck that apples are "abundance," artichokes "forgiveness," avocados "healing," and broccoli "growth." Sixty Spirit channeled fruits, vegetables, herbs, nuts, and spices with words that explain their meaning, not just spiritually, but also scientifically were gaining traction worldwide. A new bridge of intuitive food therapy was emerging, and it worked.

Time to step into my life's purpose. I'm ready Freddie.

I was destined for a wider road leading everywhere and food was the guide. As long as I can remember, I've been a crazy combo of "woo and world." A fourth-generation intuitive who played with tarot and oracle cards as a kid while others in the neighborhood were playing Crazy Eights and Go Fish. I was different and knew it. I grew up with a single, hippy mom. Other families had two parents and went to church. We went to metaphysical bookstores and got readings, burned sage, and meditated. It was evident I was a bit "left of center," and this was all I knew.

In college, I studied food science, taking deep dives into the chemistry of consumption, learning how calcium builds up into gallstones, how oils have different cooking temperatures, and how gas chromatography/ mass spectrometry measures the chemicals in food. Yep, I was a bonafide science geek, needing to know how everything worked, especially as it related to nutrition and healing. That was 35 years ago.

Around that college period when I had my eyes on a microscope, I was also working part-time for one of Hollywood's top vegetarian chefs, allowing me to enjoy my food passions and esoteric values. The Chefs were pretty spiritual, and I honed in on "cooking with consciousness" and the nuances of intuitive food prep. One never knows how a moment (or more) in one's life leads to one's purpose and dharma.

It would be several decades of life learning before I'd bring food-healing wisdom, intuition, spirituality, and practicality into a form that answered my questions about nutrition and intuition. I knew there was more to learn.

What foods are specific to my needs, wants, and desires?

How do I trust my intuition to tell me what my body needs?

Which foods raise my vibration or bring me down?

Why don't I follow the advice I give others?

I knew the answers were far more than "Sugar is bad, vegetables are good." Foods with ingredients I can't pronounce break my body down, while foods with fewer ingredients are better.

I gained and lost weight often. I tried every diet trend known to mankind. I exercised like crazy and then burned out or got injured. Rinse, cycle, repeat.

While being educated and intuitive were great combined skill sets, I was human and faced body image issues that needed attention for my self-esteem and mental health. This saga wasn't mine alone, as I commiserated with my clients about the same challenges.

Go back to your roots. You've been given a lineage and education that has the answers.

Energy, frequency, vibration—my favorite trio. I ate these words for breakfast, lunch and dinner. I enjoyed them as a delicious snack. They make up everything and provide a compass to steer my course correctly.

I reveled in the work of the late Dr. Emoto Masaru's (1943-2014) New York Times bestselling book, *Messages in Water*. He believed human consciousness could affect the molecular structure of water. He showed microscopic slides of droplets with the energy of "love" and "hate" associated with them. The water had a snowflake shape and different crystalline structures from one word to the other. There was a remarkable shift. I was intrigued to understand more.

If water's structure is altered by the energy, frequency, and vibration of words, and food is made mostly of water, then foods with words will also have an energetic shift. You have my attention Spirit.

More ingredients were needed to perfect this recipe that was swirling in my mind. Enter Dr. David Hawkins, M.D, Ph.D. (1927- 2012). Hawkins was renowned as a pioneering researcher and created the Map of Consciousness, a vibrational scale of frequency and color. The scale indicated that words had a lower to higher frequency value. "Hate' had a vibration of one hundred, while "Love" had a frequency of eight hundred. How one thinks, behaves (and thus, in my opinion), eats, has a measure of vibration. I lit up like a Christmas tree.

If I was in a bad mood or a lower vibrational state, I didn't eat well. When all were unicorns and rainbows (a higher vibrational state), I made better choices for my body. Dr. Hawkins had my fascination, and so did the nudge from Mother Nature to put this puzzle together and see how it all related to food and wellness.

So, I looked further at Mother Earth's clues with her foods that resembled the body parts they helped.

Walnuts > *Brains*

Carrots and blueberries > *Eyes*

Celery > *Bones*

Grapes > *Lungs*

Mushrooms > *Ears*

Red kidney beans > *Kidneys*

I tuned into my knowledge of the body's chakra system, the energy around color, and my passion for nature's five elements (earth, air, fire, water, and spirit), to come up with a methodology that was both spiritual and scientific. I shared these concepts with a fellow foodie and oracle, joined forces, and in 2019, The Food Healing Oracle Deck® was born.

With this progressive creation, opening up to the greater messages of food has created community, health, and expansion in my life and so many others. I can choose ahead of time what I want to shop for by using The Food Healing Deck®'s "advice" to light the way and provide an intuitive direction to higher vibrational choices.

I found the connection to infinite nourishment. If I feed myself well, I can give from the positive overflow to others. My body is a temple and will support me when I fuel it with the energy it desires.

It's my goal that each one of you becomes a Food Oracle, one who listens to Spirit's guidance for enlightenment, longevity, and wellness. You are the decider of what, when, how, and why you consume foods that matter. Make them high vibrational, and trust that your intuition knows you best!

THE TOOL

SOUL SHOPPING FOR GROCERIES

Everyone engages in shopping for meals. Many shop for the week ahead, others for the next few days, and some prefer to shop daily and stay present in the moment to what their bodies are calling for. As you become more attuned to knowing what your body needs, you'll find that you'll shop more frequently and honor the *real-time* requirements your mind, body, and soul desire.

PRESENCE IS KEY BEFORE YOU BEGIN TO SHOP

(This may be in your car before entering the store)

Before you begin your journey to the outer aisles, spend time in present awareness to clear the mind space of any clutter on your mental to-do list or thoughts of where you're to be next.

Take time to go within and connect to the needs of your soul. Here's an invocation to help you step in.

"Father-Mother God, I divinely ask to clear the space within to allow my soul to guide my nourishment needs in this now moment. I ask for the highest good of all concerned to be shown the greatest vibrational match to my body, clearing away any distractions or incongruent choices that no longer serve me. I ask for the greatest frequency of foods to be presented for my emotional, mental, physical, and spiritual (EMPS) wellness that fortifies and satisfies me on all levels. And so it is."

Next, follow your intuition to the produce section. The outer aisles are where the food is most fresh and nutritious for the body. The inner aisles are where the packaged goods are and have many preservatives to keep a longer shelf life. Remember, you are the spiritual warrior who wants foods that sustain you right now, not in future months or years, as some foods loaded with preservatives will do.

Take a look around. What do you see? What colors are striking a tone? Notice the array of herbs available. What calls to you? Breathe in the scents of nature. What do you smell? Happiness, joy, pleasure? Health, opportunity, and change? Look around. This is the medicine cabinet of life. You're being shown exactly what you need to create and manifest a meal that matters.

Notice the shapes of food—circles, ovals, spheres. What appeals? Notice the foods that invoke an emotional resonance. What are they? Why are they calling you? Tune in and listen. Connect to your body's infinite wisdom. It has served you well and will continue to every time.

Now that you've chosen your produce, it's time to consider your protein choices. How and what protein you choose is a personal choice that can only be determined by you. With The Food Healing Oracle Deck®, we focus on plant-based choices for protein. Look around and see how you feel to fortify yourself. Let your body tell you; let it be known. When you see a protein that lights up, ask yourself "Is _____ in alignment for me?" You fill in what that blank is. Your body will know. Access your intuitive wisdom.

What your body calls for may be different from one moment to the next, just like your moods. Choose accordingly now, without judgment. Make an honest choice.

If you're not getting a clear, intuitive hit, consider additional spiritual tools such as a physical pendulum, human pendulum sway test, or muscle testing. To learn more about these testing techniques, please read my blog: "Testing Techniques to Enlighten Your Food Choices" at https://centerforintuitivefoodtherapy.com/blog/

Once you have chosen your nourishment, it's time to create a perfect meal, knowing that you are aligned with your body's highest vibrational choice for this moment. If you have a copy of *The Food Healing Oracle*

Deck®, you will have a wonderful tool to help connect to your body and tune into what it's yearning for.

To keep you on your cosmic roadmap to conscious eating, I invite you to take in this sacred activation by reading below and listening to the audio version at: https://CenterForIntuitiveFoodTherapy.com/Activation

ACTIVATION

"Welcome one, welcome all. Thank you for choosing this moment to activate the connection of human doing to soul being. You are being asked to uplift and sanctify your temple with the highest vibration of nourishment at a time your body is going through a crystalline change.

As you move through dense to more buoyant frequencies and release the trappings of the earthly plane, you are asked to step further into your ascended state. You are being called to be more and do more to deepen your connection with self and understand the relationship of feeding your mind, body, and spirit with foods that not only sustain but enhance, expand, uplevel, and create a new level of awareness in your temple, one of wholeness and oneness with the totality of who you are – a Divine, interplanetary light traveler who is traversing this physical realm through your body in form and becoming one with the higher energetic being of that where you came from and that where you're going. To fortify your longevity while you are here, you are required to take care and concern of your body at the utmost level and that is up to you to make the choices that are for your highest good.

You have a pivotal role to play and that is why you are here at this moment, during a time where Mother Nature is transitioning into a utopian existence and you are being reminded that in order to have a peaceful exterior and greater vibrational surroundings, you need to have one within and that starts and ends with how and what you consume.

For you, dear one, are Nature and you are sure to be in alignment with her five elements as you eat as close to the natural ways of the land. When you become in resonance with all beings and honoring of your own temple, then you will begin to flow with greater ease, comfort, and health. Then, you will begin to open up your energy centers even further and spin with greater vibrancy so you can then offer that energy to others as well as magnetize and manifest that energy back to you.

Take a deep breath in and let it out. Again. This time breathe in your willingness to listen to your body's desires and breathe out any resistance to change. Breathe in your acceptance of eating lighter and brighter, and breathe out any impulses or cravings that no longer serve you.

Envision a golden light from Mother Earth's core coming up through your feet and entering your body—in your bones, muscles, circulatory system, and chakras. Activate the divine spark up through your crown and up to the cosmos. See a Merkaba of light spinning within and out to the Universe. See radiance glowing in all your being. Know that you are an emissary of light and are ready for this rise in consciousness and vibration.

You are able to choose the foods your body deserves with greater purpose, intention, and connection. These are the ones that will provide sustenance, healing, calm, peace, love and joy. You have a road map and a compass. It's already built inside. Allow Spirit to guide the way. The messages will come. Now, bring your attention to your third eye, located above your nose and between your eyebrows. Tap it three times. Envision a body that is strong, vital, and fluid. Ask your body what it wants to show you, tell you, and requires to allow greater harmony within the cells for communication and repair. Thank it for being so clear. For having the clarity of vision allows you to have a direct understanding that is unique to your body form and no one else's. Each body is sovereign and deserves to be honored and revered. This is your time to connect back into your body temple and love it like never before.

Make this the turning point you've been waiting for. Make this the time when you choose to nourish your body temple with intention so it can nourish you, too. In turn, you'll be able to fuel yourself with higher vibrations so you can pass this inner and ancient wisdom to your family, community, clients, and beyond for generations to come. After all, we are one. We are nature. We are Divine. We are love. We are nourished in infinitely magnificent ways. Namaste. Aho. Amen.

And so it is. . .

To your infinite wellness,

Sevante

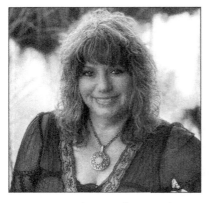

Lainie Sevante Wulkan is Founder of The Center for Intuitive Food Therapy™ (CIFT), Nourish Your Soul Ayurveda & Nourish Your Soul Retreats. She's a multi–modality healer with advanced certifications in Food Healing, Theta Healing, and EFT/Tapping. She holds a BS in Food Science, Dietetics, and Nutrition from California State University Northridge and was top of class in Jeff Primack's "Conquering All Disease Advanced Food Healing" Instructor program. She's an International bestselling Author of *The Food Healing Oracle Deck*®–*Nourishing Wisdom from Mother Earth* (Co-Authored Vol. 1 and 2 and is writing Volume 3); *Smoothies–Nourishing Wisdom Beyond the Blend, Top Exotic Foods for Natural Healing*. She also wrote a chapter for *The Energy Healers Oracle*, deemed #21 out of 100 best healing books of all time by Book Authority. Sevante is now launching the highly-anticipated seven-volume series *Feeding Your Chakras* and co-authoring *Angelic Resonance* with International Bestselling Author Angela Orora Medway–Smith.

Sevante elevates humanity by nourishing the mind, body, and soul. Her passion is felt throughout all her creations. She offers a deeper knowledge of Spirit and self-expansion to her community to have optimum emotional, mental, physical, and spiritual (EMPS) wellness.

She travels globally with Nourish Your Soul Retreats, speaks at holistic festivals worldwide, teaches online classes to become a Certified Intuitive Food Therapist, offers private readings and healing sessions, hosts the Nourish Your Soul Show, and is expanding her Ayurvedic tea and incense imports from Nepal across USA and Canada.

Sevante is nestled on a beautiful island in Southwest Florida with her husband, music producer Howard Merlin Wulkan, and their four-legged brood amongst palm trees, enchanted ponds, peacocks, and the best of Mother Nature's bounty.

CIFT:
https://centerforintuitivefoodtherapy.com/

Nourish Your Soul Retreats:
https://www.facebook.com/groups/nourishyoursoulretreats

Nourish Your Soul Ayurveda:
https://www.facebook.com/nourishyoursoultea

Nourish Your Soul Show:
https://www.facebook.com/nourishyoursoulshow

CHAPTER 2

THE REAL FOUNTAIN OF YOUTH

LEARN MY SECRET
TO STAYING YOUNG FOREVER

Vito Kostrzewski, Ph.D.

MY STORY

Have you ever been intrigued by the secret of the fountain of youth? I've spent most of my adult life wanting to stay young forever. Why? Because I hate getting old, weak, and frail and being unable to do my favorite sports and activities. When I go to the doctor's office and see all the old people who can hardly move, is that the future I'm looking forward to? Is that where I'm heading?

My answer was a solid no, and that's why I needed to find a way to avoid it. That was the main reason why I was fascinated with the idea of cracking the code of the fountain of youth.

It took me years of research and testing until I finally cracked the code. As a scientist with a Ph.D. in materials engineering, I learned how to research and determine what information is useful and what information is useless (and needs to be disregarded). I went through a tough period of several years right after the real estate market crash in Florida when I couldn't afford it and therefore didn't have health insurance. I dealt with sciatica and later a leaky gut and joint problems. I conducted thorough research and applied the suggestions. They worked well and I eliminated these problems.

Later, when I had health insurance and doctor's visits and tests paid for by the insurance company, I still had to do my research. I was very unhappy with the suggestions given to me by traditional doctors, which required me to take plenty of pills with bad side effects and/or undergo surgery. I studied articles and books written by alternative and functional doctors like Dr. Al Sears, Dr. Mark Hyman, Dr. Michael T. Murray, Dr. Keith Scott-Mumby, Dr. Fred Pescatore, Dr. Mark Stengler, and Dr. Marc Micozzi. I tested their suggestions and recommendations on myself and, later, on my girlfriend.

I'm currently free of any chronic diseases, my test results are normal and in range, and I feel like I'm 15-25 years younger. That's like drinking from the Fountain of Youth! I'll show you how you can achieve the same state of great health and feel fantastic if you follow my recommendations.

Several longevity markers determine our biological age, which deteriorates as we age. Slowing down, stopping, and reversing that deterioration is the key to the Fountain of Youth. So, what are these markers, and what can we do to slow down, stop, and even reverse the deterioration?

The first marker is our telomeres. Their length determines our biological age. As we age, they get shorter and shorter. The shorter they are, the sicker we become, and eventually, they'll become so short that we die.

The next marker is our stem cells; their quality deteriorates, and their number decreases as we age.

Then, the mitochondria, whose quality and quantity determine our biological age.

The state of our blood vessels, especially our arteries, also affects our biological age. Plugged-up arteries reduce the flow of nutrients and oxygen to our organs, causing rapid deterioration.

There are five steps leading to the Fountain of Youth. The first two steps are the foundation on which the remaining three steps will be built.

THE TOOL

5 STEPS TO THE FOUNTAIN OF YOUTH

1. **Mastering mindset.**
2. **Elimination of all chronic diseases and restoring the body to a healthy state.**
3. **Slowing down the biological clock.**
4. **Stopping the biological clock.**
5. **Reversing the biological clock.**

Let's examine all the steps and the ways to achieve them.

1. MASTERING THE MINDSET

The key to a good mental state is to keep a positive attitude most of the time, be grateful for everything that we possess and receive, and have high self-esteem and a high level of self-confidence. I added daily affirmations to improve my mindset like: I feel great, I feel fantastic, I'm young forever, I'm healthy, I'm strong, etc. You can add any positive affirmations that you like.

Physical activities also have a great influence on the state of our mind. They cause the brain to calm down and release more serotonin, which is a pleasure hormone. That increases our feeling of well-being. I feel very calm and relaxed after my exercise, especially when I add a sauna session at the end.

2. ELIMINATION OF ALL CHRONIC DISEASES AND RESTORING THE BODY TO A HEALTHY STATE

What are the most dangerous chronic diseases that kill the most people in the US? Heart diseases, including cardiovascular problems, kill almost 700 thousand people a year, and the number keeps growing. The next one is cancer, killing over 600 thousand people a year, and the number is growing every year.

Those two main killers are followed by chronic lower respiratory diseases, stroke, Alzheimer's disease, diabetes, and chronic liver and kidney diseases. We're also plagued by other debilitating, although not deadly, diseases like dementia, arthritis, obesity, malfunction of joints, hormonal imbalances, sarcopenia, osteoporosis, digestive, eye, and sleep disorders, etc.

What are the main contributors to these diseases? It's the lifestyle, the environment, and elevated internal inflammation. These three contributors are interconnected.

Our lifestyle covers our environment, what we eat, what we do, what we use on our bodies, and what we find around us. Our environment covers the area surrounding us, including the people around us.

Internal inflammation is primarily caused by energetic and physical toxins. Examples of energetic toxins include excessive stress, interactions with negative people, listening to negative news, etc. Physical toxins come primarily from items that we ingest, like synthetic drugs (most prescribed drugs are synthetic), microplastics from plastic packaging and plastic bottles, processed foods, veggies and fruits containing pesticides, insecticides, and heavy metals, GMOs, meats containing antibiotics, and hormones, foods laden with sugar or carbs that easily convert into sugar, and from items that we apply to our bodies like cosmetics, make-up, etc. Internal inflammation can also be caused by physical trauma, injuries, and surgeries that aren't healing quickly and cause the immune system to overreact and by infections with bacteria and viruses that were not treated quickly.

Let's start with the main killing diseases: heart failure and cardiovascular disorders. The most frequent reason for heart failure is a heart attack, also called a myocardial infarction. It occurs when the blood flow to the heart gets blocked, either by a clot, a spasm of the coronary artery, or an accumulation of plaque. Blood delivers oxygen and nutrients to the heart muscle so if their flow gets stopped, the heart muscle dies very quickly. The heart can also deteriorate due to problems with the heart muscle; however, most heart problems are caused by heavy plaque in the arteries. Bad arteries in the heart mean there are also bad arteries leading to main organs (like the brain, lungs, liver, and kidney) often causing deterioration and failure of these organs.

We've all heard the expression of hardening of the arteries or arteriosclerosis. They describe a condition in which a hardened grease called plaque gets stuck to the walls of the arteries, causing its interior diameter to narrow down and restrict the blood flow. When the restriction becomes 90 percent or more, it becomes life-threatening.

Although big pharma blames it on high cholesterol, multiple recent studies showed that cholesterol was not the culprit. Most of our cholesterol is produced by our liver and it's used by our body to make important hormones like estrogen and testosterone and to protect our neurons in the brain. HDL cholesterol helps remove plaque from the arteries. Recent research found that the main culprit was homocysteine. Its elevated levels are caused by high inflammation and are also a major contributor to all chronic diseases listed above. Another test for internal inflammation is to measure the level of C-reactive protein. The natural way to reduce the homocysteine level is to take natural B-Complex, trimethylglycine (TMG), and l-serine supplements.

What can we do to reduce the risk of a heart attack due to plugged-up arteries? The first step is to reduce the level of internal inflammation in our body and detox from heavy metals and toxic chemicals. The internal inflammation can be lowered by taking popular supplements like turmeric (the active component is called curcumin) with added black pepper extract (BioPerine) to improve absorption, ginger root extract and boswellia serrata also known as frankincense. All of them come in the form of capsules.

For detoxification, we can use EDTA Chelation applied intravenously or through ingestion, modified citrus pectin in capsule form, or detox formulas based on mostly fermented fruits and veggies in powder form.

The next step is to clean up the arteries. The best combo consists of vitamin C, preferably the liposomal version for improved absorption, vitamin D3, vitamin K2-MK7, and magnesium, preferably in the form of chelate, glycinate, or citrate to improve the absorption. To improve and speed up this process, proteolytic enzymes like Nattokinase or Lumbrokinase are recommended, which mostly dissolve and remove fibrins, which are also part of the plaque. Dirty arteries can lead to high blood pressure (HBP) that can lead to stroke and failure of other major organs like the heart, liver, and kidneys. Another contributing factor to the HBP is the hardening of the arteries as the levels of nitric oxide (NO) decrease with age. To stop and reverse the decline of NO, functional doctors recommend taking NO generators like l-arginine, l-citrulline, and Omega-3 oils containing DHA and EPA.

Stroke is brain damage caused by stopping blood flow in the blood vessel or by rapture of a blood vessel, causing blood flooding of surrounding areas. When blood stops flowing, nerves in the brain die very rapidly. When blood floods certain areas of the brain, it results in paralysis of the limbs and organs which the brain area controls.

To strengthen the heart muscle, functional doctors recommend coenzyme Q-10, the Ubiquinol version for increased absorption, l-carnitine, and hawthorn berry. The most important step is switching to a healthy diet consisting of a blend of meat or wild-caught fish, vegetables, fruits, and slow carbs that are preferably organic and incorporating exercise, preferably HIIT (High-Intensity Interval Training) like PACE Express developed by Dr. Sears that takes less than 16 minutes to do.

The next main killing disease is cancer. What's the best way to prevent cancer? A healthy and balanced diet, frequent detoxing from heavy metals and chemicals, plenty of exercise, and stress relieving activities. We also need to strengthen our immune system by taking intravenous or liposomal vitamin C, vitamin D3, E, A, selenium, monolaurin, colostrum, beta-glucans, and antioxidants: glutathione, coenzyme Q-10.

What do we need to eliminate other chronic diseases? The main contributors to all of them are internal inflammation and an unhealthy lifestyle consisting of poor diet and lack of motion and exercise. A poor diet is full of processed foods, Omega-6 rich oils, quick carbs like sugar, wheat products, and corn, and lacking healthy vegetables and fruits. An example of a healthy diet is the Mediterranean diet.

The best type of exercise is HIIT which strengthens our respiratory and cardiovascular system. It consists of periods of high and low intensity. Good sports for that are football, basketball, ice hockey, tennis, racquetball, and pickleball which mix up high and low-intensity periods.

3. SLOWING DOWN THE BIOLOGICAL CLOCK

We have three main markers showing our biological age: telomeres, stem cells, and mitochondria.

Telomeres are a little bit of genetic material at the end of a DNA strand like aglets, which are the little pieces of hard plastic at the ends of shoelaces. Their length determines our biological age, the shorter they are the older we are.

The enzyme that controls the length of telomeres is called telomerase. By increasing the amount of telomerase, we can slow down the decline, stop the decline, and reverse the decline of telomeres.

The best telomerase boosters are the herb astragalus, plenty of magnesium (600-1000mg/day), high level of HDL, HIIT, low levels of homocysteine which is the main contributor to heart failure, low levels of chemicals, and high levels of Omega-3 compounds (DHA and EPA). Vitamins C, D3, E, B1, and B12 also increase telomerase levels.

The next biological age marker is stem cells. Their quality and quantity decline with time, making us biologically older. When we get older, our stem cells are less active and in smaller numbers, so it takes much longer to heal any injury.

Stem cells deteriorate quicker in the presence of chronic inflammation, elevated levels of toxins from food, cosmetics, air, smoking, poor diet, obesity, and excessive stress.

We can boost the number and quality of stem cells by eating fresh blueberries which are known to contain resveratrol, green tea extract (EGCG), l-carnosine, NAD+, vitamins D3, B9, B12, getting plenty of sleep, and using hyperbaric chambers with pure oxygen (HBOT) to deliver more oxygen to all cells.

The third main marker of biological aging is mitochondria. Mitochondria are the little furnaces contained in most cells that generate energy for the body by burning ATP (obtained from glucose) in oxygen. Children and teenagers have thousands of mitochondria in each cell, so they are full of energy, can run forever, and don't feel cold. Old people have only a few mitochondria left in each cell; they get tired very quickly and are cold-sensitive.

We can slow down and stop the decline of mitochondria by providing them with special nutrients. Nutrients for increasing mitochondrial energy production are acetyl-l-carnitine (ALC), coenzyme Q-10 (Co Q-10), alpha lipoic acid, preferably in the R form (r-ALA), cordyceps, Rhodiola rosea, astaxanthin and l-carnitine, preferably as l-carnitine tartrate or propionyl l-carnitine as they are more absorbable. To regenerate mitochondria, we can take taurine, magnesium as malate, chelate, glycinate or citrate, and niacin in the form of niacinamide and nicotinic acid. To regrow mitochondria, we take pyrroloquinoline quinone (PQQ), resveratrol, preferably as trans-resveratrol, pomegranate extract, green tea extract, ashwagandha extract, and gynostemma extract.

Before we can move to the next step, which is stopping the biological clock, we need to optimize several systems in our body: the digestive system, detoxification system, hormonal system, immune system, and the state of our bones, joints, and muscles.

Our digestive system controls the absorption of all the nutrients we ingest. We can take all the nutrients we need, but if they don't get absorbed into our blood, they're useless. Most of our immune system is located around our small intestine, so problems with the digestive system create problems with the immune system.

The detoxification system consists of the food elimination system located in the large intestine, liver, kidneys, lymphatic system, and skin. We must keep these components in good condition because if any of them malfunction, more and more toxins accumulate in the blood and poison our bodies.

The hormonal system consists of thyroid hormones, adrenal hormones, and sex hormones.

Thyroid hormones control our metabolism. When the thyroid slows down, everything slows down, resulting in fatigue, weight gain, depression, memory loss, low sex drive, elevated cholesterol, and heart, skin, nails, and digestive system problems. We need to supplement it with natural thyroid hormones, preferably a blend of T4 and T3. A healthy thyroid needs plenty of l-tyrosine, iodine, vitamins: C, D, E, B-Complex, iron, zinc, and selenium.

Adrenal hormones, which are cortisol and DHEA, are very important to our health. DHEA gets converted to estrogen and testosterone. Low levels of DHEA lead to cardiovascular disease, autoimmune disorders, weight gain, diabetes, sexual dysfunction, and lower immune response. Cortisol contributes to fighting infection, stabilizing blood sugar, use of nutrients, and responding to higher stress.

Important sex hormones are testosterone, especially for men, and estrogen and progesterone, especially for women. To stay healthy, men need plenty of testosterone and a little bit of estrogen and progesterone. Women need an equal amount of estrogen and progesterone and a little bit of testosterone.

The main bone disease is osteoporosis which causes loss of bone strength due to loss of mineral content and collagen. Osteoporosis affects mostly older people, especially women. To prevent and combat osteoporosis, we should take magnesium, calcium, vitamin K2-MK7, D3, and collagen and balance our sex hormones.

It's a known fact that muscle tissue shrinks as we age. This process is called sarcopenia, and it's primarily caused by a decreased metabolic rate and lack of strength training. To stop and reverse this process, we need to increase our mitochondrial function and supply our body with proper nutrients, such as amino acids needed to build new muscle, Vitamin D3, K2, calcium, magnesium, and exercise, especially weight training.

Exercise, including weight training, is also an important element of keeping our joints healthy. Our joints also need proper nutrients to function and rebuild, such as curcumin, Boswellia serrata, MSM (methylsulfonylmethane) which is organic sulfur, glucosamine, and hyaluronic acid which is the main component in the lubricant in the joint.

4. AND 5. STOPPING AND REVERSING THE BIOLOGICAL CLOCK

These steps are just the natural progression from Chapter 3 after we optimize our systems and incorporate all suggestions, including proper nutrition.

To stay healthy, we need to have a healthy lifestyle consisting of a healthy diet, exercise, including HIIT and weight training, detox, including detoxifying supplements and saunas, mitochondrial support, including supplements and cold treatments like cold showers and cold plunges, HBOT to increase our oxygen intake, good sex as it's beneficial to our mental and physical health, a positive attitude, relaxation, and gratitude.

A good choice of supplements includes a complete multivitamin with minerals, Vitamin C, D3, K2-MK7, B-Complex, Omega-3 oils, magnesium, zinc, selenium, boron, NAD+, quercetin, luteolin, hesperidin, resveratrol, pterostilbene, turmeric/curcumin with Bioperine, EGCG, branched amino acids, ALC, n-acetylcysteine (NAC), PQQ, r-ALA, ashwagandha, astaxanthin, phosphatidylcholine, gingko biloba, l-carnosine, l-citrulline, l-arginine, TMG and for the eye support: bilberry, lutein and zeaxanthin.

I tested all the above-listed recommendations on myself and so far, I achieved great results as I enjoy great health, mobility, and strength of a healthy man 15-25 years younger than I am.

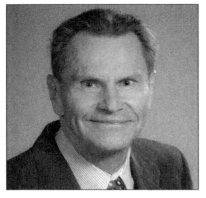

Vito Kostrzewski was born and grew up in Warsaw, Poland. I started my studies in Chemical Engineering at the Warsaw Polytechnic and received a government scholarship to continue my studies in Germany where I graduated with a M.S. degree in Chemical Engineering. Subsequently, I received a scholarship from the University of Pittsburgh to continue graduate studies there where I graduated with a Ph.D. degree in Materials Engineering specializing in plastics processing.

I worked for over 19 years for medium, large, and giant companies as a polymer scientist holding engineering and technical management positions.

In 2003, I moved to Cape Coral, acquired a real estate license, and became a real estate agent and real estate investor. I continue working as a Realtor and have been awarded the prestigious award of the 5 Star Real Estate Agent by Gulfshore Life for 10 years in a row.

I used my knowledge of chemistry and materials to extensively study alternative medicine which helped me recover from sciatica and other problems. I developed effective techniques to keep my health in peak condition and highly reduced the chances of getting any chronic diseases.

As a trained scientist in Materials Engineering, I learned a lot about the other side of the world, which is the energy world. I expanded my studies into energy healing, learned several techniques for using energy in healing, and became a certified Theta Healing Practitioner.

For most of my adult life, I have been fascinated with staying young and healthy and with the Fountain of Youth and I've continued with my research in this area.

If you have any questions about staying in great health and slowing down the aging process, connect with me:

Phone: 239.910.5400

Email: vitohealth@vitofl.com

CHAPTER 3

FAITH UNBROKEN

TRANSFORMING ADVERSITY THROUGH WORDS, BELIEF, AND RESILIENCE

Karen Rudolf

MY STORY

Tuning Into Tranquility: The High Vibrational Healing Method

In the silence that follows the storm, where do we find the strength to whisper to the shadows, "I see you, and I am not afraid?"

My life has been a tapestry of interconnected events and moments that seem both chaotic and divinely ordered, leading me to ask: What binds these threads together? Is it the search for meaning, the longing for connection, or perhaps the discovery that in our most solitary struggles, I am, in fact, most deeply connected to the world around me?

This is a tale of such discovery, a journey from the depths of solitude and pain to the peaks of understanding and unity. It's a story not just about finding myself but also about reconnecting with the universal heartbeat that pulses through us all.

In the labyrinth of life's unexpected twists, two profound events unfolded like dark, unfurling blossoms, each petal revealing shadows and, ultimately, leading to light.

My journey through emotional turmoil and physical trials became the unlikely prelude to self-discovery and a re-defined sense of purpose. Herein lies the tale of that transformation, marked first by the heartache of divorce and then by a harrowing accident in a land far from home.

DIVORCE AS A PRELUDE TO SELF-DISCOVERY

The end of my marriage was not just the closing of a chapter but the tearing of a map I was using to navigate the world. Left in the wake of divorce were fragments of identity and shards of dreams we built together. I lost my sense of identity within the marriage, and once resolved, I felt alone, naked, and exposed. The initial feelings of loss and disorientation enveloped me like a dense fog, making the familiar seem foreign and the future unfathomable. Bottom line, I was scared shitless, not just for myself, what was to become of our daughters, who were stuck in the middle of the chaotic swirl and ongoing battling. It very much saddened me, and I felt helpless and stuck.

In this chasm of despair, I confronted my deepest fears and insecurities, questioning not just the fabric of my relationship but the very essence of my being. A fleeting moment of suicide crossed my thoughts. I felt my life was over. Who was I beyond the roles I played for others for so long? The answer lay hidden, buried under years of compromise and forgotten dreams.

Yet, it was in the deepest night of the soul that a flicker of understanding began to emerge. This end could be a beginning—a harsh but honest foundation upon which I could rebuild, not just my life but myself. The realization dawned slowly that this rupture offered a rare opportunity: to embark on the most significant journey of all, the journey within. It was a chance to discover my desires, my values, and my strength, unencumbered by another's expectations.

THE ACCIDENT IN COSTA RICA

The quest for self-discovery took an unexpected detour years later when, seeking solace and adventure in the lush landscapes of Costa Rica, fate intervened with a dramatic lesson in vulnerability and resilience. The day began with the promise of adventure, the tropical sun casting a golden glow over the verdant jungle that stretched out to touch the azure skies. A horseback ride along the secluded beaches of Marbella was meant to be a balm for my bruised spirit, a step towards reclaiming joy and freedom.

But as the horse and I moved as one, navigating the uneven terrain that led to the sea, a sudden shift turned tranquility into chaos. In a heartbeat, the animal spun around, and I was flung into the air, time stretching out as I fell toward the unforgiving earth below.

Lying on the sand, the initial shock gave way to a raw, primal fear as I realized the severity of my situation. I thought I'd panic. However, I was calm; everything appeared in slow motion. I was in shock. Pain coursed through my body, a stark testament to my fragility. The isolation of being in a foreign country, unable to communicate my pain or navigate the path forward, compounded the terror. The vulnerability of this moment laid bare all illusions of control I thought I wielded over life. *Will I ever walk again?* Fear rushed through me.

Yet, amidst the swirling panic and pain, a deeper awareness began to crystallize in the moment. *How will I get home?* I couldn't move my lower body at all, and my support system was so far away. This accident, much like my divorce, was not just a trial to endure but a call to awaken. It demanded surrender to the moment, trust in the unseen forces that guide our journey, and the courage to face the unknown with an open heart. The realization that I was about to embark on a profound journey of healing and self-discovery, powered by an inner strength I was only just beginning to understand, became a beacon of hope in the darkest night.

These catalysts, each an ordeal in its own right, forged a path through the wilderness of my soul, leading me not to answers but to better questions, questions that would compel me to dive deeper, reach higher, and ultimately, find a truer reflection of myself in the still waters of introspection and renewal. I began reflecting on all I'd learned and who I'd become over the years as a result. *What are my first steps? Who can I ask to support me as the team player I've been trained as?* I began focusing on my healing and turned over the baton to others to be of support in getting me back to the States.

In the sterile, white expanse of a Costa Rican hospital room post-surgery, far removed from the familiarity of home, I found myself enveloped in a cocoon of solitude. The accident had not only fractured my body but also stripped away the bustling noise of everyday life, leaving me in a forced retreat within the confines of my own mind. The language barrier erected a wall between me and the world outside, each failed attempt at communication a stark reminder of my isolation. As I stared out the window, I saw a mountain. I looked down at my immobile feet, barely moving a toe. Looking back at the mountainside, I remember thinking, how do you transverse a mountain? In a moment, it came to me with the faith of a mustard seed. *One foot in front of another.*

Physical pain became a constant companion, its sharp reminders punctuating my days and nights, challenging my resolve, and forcing me to confront the fragility of my existence.

It was within this stillness of solitude and reflection that constant questions surfaced: *Will I walk again? Can I? Will I? What will my life be like after this?* It seemed like a distant chance that I embarked on the most profound journey of my life—the journey within. The silence, punctuated only by the distant echoes of footsteps and the intermittent beeps of machines, became the backdrop for a deep, introspective dive. Questions I long avoided, buried under the debris of daily distractions, now demanded my attention. Who am I in the absence of the roles I play? What truths about myself have I ignored? How can I find peace amidst pain? These inquiries, once mere whispers, grew louder, echoing in the caverns of my mind.

This period of forced reflection became a gateway to clarity. I realized that my previous explorations into the mysteries of quantum physics and the ethereal realms of spirituality were not mere intellectual pursuits but preparations for this moment of reckoning. These studies had subtly woven a tapestry of understanding and belief that now served as my foundation in the face of adversity.

Drawing upon this reservoir of knowledge, I began to apply the principles that had fascinated me in theory to the stark reality of my situation. Visualization techniques, once practiced with the detached curiosity of a student, became vital tools in my healing arsenal. I closed my eyes and pictured my body mending; each cell rejuvenated, each bone knitting back stronger. This practice, rooted in the Law of Attraction's assertion that our thoughts shape our reality, became a daily ritual, infusing my spirit with hope and my body with the energy to heal.

Affirmations played a critical role. In moments of despair, when the pain seemed insurmountable and my situation hopeless, I would whisper to myself, "I am healing, I am strong, I am surrounded by love and light." These words, simple yet profound, became a mantra that helped me navigate through the darkest hours, a lifeline to the belief in my innate resilience and the universe's capacity for healing.

Meditation, previously a practice I engaged in sporadically, now became as essential as breathing. It offered a respite from the pain, a sanctuary of peace in the turmoil. Through meditation, I observed my thoughts and emotions without judgment and accepted my present reality while also envisioning a future of wellness and vitality. This practice deepened my connection to my inner self, to the quiet, unwavering source of strength that I neglected in the pursuit of external achievements and validation. I closed my eyes, got still, and tuned out the noise of the happenings around me. I took deep, slow breaths and slowly breathed out any toxic energy of negative thoughts. I began seeing and visualizing myself walking—breath in, breath out. Healing—breath in and breath out. I began feeling encouraged. There was hope!

This period of recovery became a profound teacher. The solitude forced upon me became a sacred space for introspection, a crucible in which my true essence was refined and revealed. The principles once learned became abstract concepts that became the pillars upon which I built my pathway to healing. They taught me that even in our most vulnerable moments, we possess the power to shape our journey, find peace amidst chaos, and emerge from the shadows with a deeper understanding of our purpose and potential. This journey within, born out of necessity, illuminated the path to a more authentic, empowered self, forever altering my course and my comprehension of life's intricate tapestry.

The twin pillars of my recovery and personal evolution emerged distinctly as the power of presence and surrender, alongside the untapped well of inner strength and the unquantifiable value of community. Each lesson wove into my narrative a richer tapestry of understanding, fundamentally altering my approach to life and its inevitable challenges.

THE POWER OF PRESENCE AND SURRENDER

In the confines of a hospital room, the future seemed distant, and the past a closed book. I was left with nothing but the present moment, a concept I had often brushed aside in the pursuit of future ambitions or shadows of past regrets. Yet, in this forced stillness, the present moment bloomed with possibilities. Pain, fear, and uncertainty became not just obstacles but invitations to deepen my engagement with the here and now.

Living in the moment taught me the essence of surrender—not as an act of defeat but as a profound acceptance of what is. This acceptance opened new pathways of healing and understanding, illuminating the intrinsic beauty and potential of the present. When I surrendered to the moment, I caught any negative thoughts that kept me from my goal of walking once more. The more I surrendered the more I became encouraged. I allowed myself to be open to the outcomes I hadn't planned or foreseen, recognizing that sometimes, what we perceive as setbacks are indeed steps forward on a path yet unseen.

To those navigating their storms, I share this insight: practice mindfulness as a gateway to presence and surrender. Start with simple breathing exercises, focusing on the inhale and exhale to anchor yourself in the now. Embrace journaling not just as a record of thoughts but as a mindfulness practice, reflecting on the current moment's textures, colors, and emotions. These practices cultivate a mindset that values the present moment as a friend, not an adversary, opening your heart to the flow of life with trust and grace.

HARNESSING INNER STRENGTH AND THE IMPORTANCE OF COMMUNITY

Throughout this journey, I discovered reserves of inner strength I never knew. This strength was not a loud, clamoring force but a quiet certainty that emerged in moments of solitude, in making peace with my vulnerabilities, and in the conscious choice to focus on healing and positivity.

Yet, this inner strength did not exist in isolation. It was amplified and nurtured by the community around me. Friends, family, and even strangers across the globe became beacons of support, their words and thoughts weaving a net of collective strength that held me when I faltered. Something as simple as getting to the bathroom and wiping myself—my children and bestie reminded me it was temporary. *Will it be?* It was humiliating enough that I was in diapers and couldn't even wipe myself. *Surrender to what is!* I had no control of what I had no control of.

My girlfriend created a Go-Fund-Me account, and my former teammates came together, forming an even larger team to make calls and speak with embassies. WhatsApp became my connection to the world beyond, and my Facebook page blew up each day with well-wishers. Many commented that they wouldn't have known what they'd do in my situation. The number of messages blew me away. This experience underscored the importance of community—not just as a social construct but as a vital source of healing and empowerment.

Building or leaning into your community doesn't require grand gestures. Start with openness—sharing your journey, your struggles, and your victories. Engage with support groups to connect with others on similar paths. Volunteer your time or expertise, fostering a spirit of giving that often returns to you tenfold. Remember, every interaction is an opportunity to strengthen the bonds of community, offering support and receiving it in turn.

The lessons of presence, surrender, inner strength, and community are not just pillars for recovery but for life itself. They teach us that every moment is a gift, that acceptance opens the door to new possibilities, that we possess untold reserves of strength, and that in our interconnectedness lies our greatest power. Once embraced, these principles illuminate a path not just to healing but to a deeper, more connected way of living.

Embarking on a journey of self-discovery and healing can be transformative, yet knowing where to start is often the biggest hurdle. Through my own path of recovery and reflection, I've found solace and strength in practices that ground me in the present and foster a deep sense of gratitude and connection. Here, I share with you the practical wisdom that has illuminated my way, hoping it will do the same for you.

THE TOOL

GUIDED MEDITATION FOR HEALING

1. *Find a Quiet Space*
   Choose a comfortable and quiet place where you won't be disturbed. Sit or lie down in a comfortable position.

2. *Breathe Deeply:*
   Close your eyes and take a deep breath through your nose, allowing your stomach to expand fully. Exhale slowly through your mouth. Repeat this deep breathing for a few minutes until you feel more relaxed.

3. *Visualize Healing:*
   Picture a warm, healing light above your head. With each inhale, visualize this light descending into your body, spreading warmth and healing energy to every part of you. Imagine the light specifically targeting areas of pain or discomfort, soothing them gently.

4. *Affirm Your Healing:*
   As you bask in this light, repeat to yourself, "With every breath, I invite healing and peace into my body. I am strong, resilient, and whole.

5. *Gradually Return:*
   After spending a few minutes in this state, slowly bring your awareness back to the present. Wiggle your fingers and toes, and when you're ready, open your eyes.

JOURNALING FOR SELF-DISCOVERY

Start with gratitude:

Begin each journaling session by listing three things you are grateful for today. This can be as simple as a sunny day, a friend's support, or something you learned about yourself.

Reflect on your journey:

Use prompts to guide your reflection. Some examples include:

- "What lesson did today teach me?"
- "When did I feel most at peace today, and why?"
- "What is one fear I faced today, and how did it make me feel?"

SET INTENTIONS:

Conclude by setting an intention for the next day. It could relate to your personal growth, how you want to treat others or a goal you wish to achieve. Daily Practices for Gratitude and Connection.

MORNING GRATITUDE:

Each morning, before you start your day, think of three things you're grateful for. This simple act sets a positive tone for the day ahead.

Acts of Kindness: Make it a point to perform at least one act of kindness each day. It could be something as small as complimenting someone, helping a neighbor, or sending a thoughtful message to a friend.

Evening Reflection: Spend a few minutes each evening reflecting on your day. Acknowledge one moment where you felt connected to someone else or something greater than yourself. This practice fosters a deep sense of belonging and reminds us of our interconnectedness.

By integrating these practices into your daily routine, you embark on a profound journey toward healing and self-discovery. Remember, the path is not about reaching a destination but about embracing each step with intention, gratitude, and open-heartedness.

This journey, a dance within the silent chambers of my soul, taught me the profound truths of resilience, healing, and the unyielding power of the human spirit. Embracing my shadows did not diminish my light but rather allowed it to shine more brightly, illuminating paths of growth and empowerment I had never imagined possible. I learned that within each of us lies an inexhaustible well of strength, ready to guide us through our darkest nights and lead us into the dawn of new beginnings.

To you, the reader, standing at the threshold of your own voyage of self-discovery, know that the dance within beckons with the promise of transformation. Your shadows are not to be feared but embraced, for they hold the keys to your deepest strength and resilience. You are more powerful than you know, more connected to the fabric of the universe than you can imagine, and fully capable of navigating the complexities of your journey.

I invite you to step into the dance of your own life with courage and openness, trusting in the rhythm of your spirit to guide you. Together, in the shared dance of humanity, we find unity and hope bound by the common threads of our experiences and dreams. May your journey be filled with growth, healing, and the discovery of the boundless potential that resides within you.

In the tapestry of life, we often find our most profound growth in the wake of challenges that test our strength and resilience. My journey, marked by personal upheaval and a life-altering accident, has been a testament to the power of inner strength, mindfulness, and the healing potential of an anti-inflammatory lifestyle. These experiences have not only shaped me but have also been the bedrock of Tranquil SOULutions, a sanctuary I founded in 2007 to guide others through their transformations.

Emerging from the depths of personal trials—a divorce that questioned my identity and a severe accident in Costa Rica that tested my physical and emotional limits—I've discovered the indispensable value of presence, surrender, and the healing power of our own thoughts and beliefs. These revelations were not mere epiphanies but beacons that lit my path to developing a unique program focused on stress alleviation and embracing an anti-inflammatory lifestyle.

This program is the culmination of my life's work and learning, designed to empower you to navigate your challenges with grace and emerge with a renewed sense of self and well-being. Through practices like guided meditation for healing, journaling for self-discovery, and daily gratitude, I invite you to embark on a journey of introspection, healing, and profound growth.

As a Life Strategist and Catalyst for Change, my mission is to guide you toward a harmonious balance in life, integrating emotional, mental, and spiritual growth with practical strategies for stress management and holistic health. If you're ready to transform your perception, tap into your inner strength, and embrace your journey with openness and courage, I am here to support you.

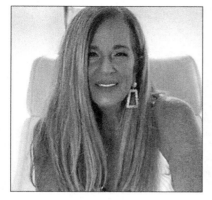

Karen Rudolf is a transformative Life Strategist, "Super Stress Reducer," and four-time international bestselling author. Founder of Tranquil SOULutions, she is dedicated to empowering personal and professional growth through a "W"holistic approach. With a background in nursing and extensive training in the 7 Pillars of Health, she empowers individuals to overcome challenges and thrive using effective communication, self-leadership, boosting self-esteem, and fostering "W"holistic well-being and decreasing stress, which results in a "W"holistic approach to personal and professional growth. Her work shifts perceptions and nurtures resilience and peace, making her a trusted guide in life's journey.

Let's connect and explore how we can walk this path together towards healing, empowerment, and a life lived with intention and joy.

https://linktr.ee/tranquilsoulutions

https://www.linkedin.com/in/tranquilsoulutions/

https://www.facebook.com/karen.rudolf.14/

https://www.instagram.com/tranquilsoulutions/

407-920-4288

https://calendly.com/tranquilsoulutions/30-minutes-meet-greet

Podcast: Awakening Potential:

https://open.spotify.com/show/4YWLGUPg3rWtumXl084oEJ

FREE GIFT: grab yours at: https://karenrudolf.com/freegiftfromkaren

CHAPTER 4

INTENTIONAL INTUITIVE CONSUMPTION

MAKING FOOD FUN (AND HEALTHY) AGAIN

Kari Bozic

MY STORY

Have you ever walked into the kitchen and thought: *Why am I here?* It's not hunger; there's not the slightest rumble in your belly.

I was feeling empty, and I didn't mean my stomach. I sensed something was missing. If I could find that one little morsel to stick in my mouth, endorphins would go off, and everything would be all better (and the void would filled), but for how long?

I've gone as far as sleep-eating. I woke in the mornings accusing family members: "I know you ate the Oreos; just admit it!" "Check your teeth," they would reply.

When I got to the mirror, I was horrified to find remnants of black cookie pieces in my teeth. I self-sabotaged in my sleep!

What the heck am I doing to myself?

A couple of years ago, I had a medical event. I woke in the middle of the night feeling I was about to be sick and ran to the bathroom, only to later awaken on the floor with a massive lump on my head. I had no idea how long I was there or what was happening. I had dizzy spells before but dismissed them, explaining them away for one reason or another, but this was different, and I was scared. Turns out I had an episode of vertigo reflux, and it most likely wasn't the first.

It was time to get serious about what I was eating and why, most importantly, what it was doing to me.

I started examining my eating habits and found a multi-step process. The first step was mindset. I recently completed a program that helped me understand that when we genuinely love, accept, and speak nicely to ourselves, many things fall into place, and we start to align with life. These teachings opened my awareness of how my body and mind communicate with each other.

The next step was to eat with intention.

I was learning to *be* with my food, not watching TV, on the phone, or reading a book. To eat using all five senses, increasing awareness of how each bite made me feel, what thoughts came to mind while I savored each bite, and then listening to my body in those next hours and days and noting how it was responding.

I found that some things I thought were healthy disagreed with me. I could tell by upset stomachs, migraines, or even inflammation in my joints—also, the mental part, the altering of my mood, or increased brain fog.

The third step was intuitive eating. I developed my intuition and learned to know when I was or wasn't in alignment with what was in front of me. I knew this by the hints my mind or body was sending. I felt my shoulders drop and my body lean away from something undesirable or a warm, internal glow that made me stand taller, eager for nourishment. As I learned this, one of the fantastic side effects was that I ate differently, craved different foods, and, as a bonus, reduced my waistline.

With each day and meal that passed, I changed. I had more energy, my mind was clearer, and I could tell how it would affect me before I put something in my mouth. I enjoyed eating and was having fun in the kitchen.

Like anything in life, you're already halfway there if you have fun.

In 2022, I was introduced to the Food Healing Oracle Deck®. Lainie, the co-creator of the cards, was a guest speaker in my empowerment group. I pre-ordered my cards to have my own set to follow along with. I had no idea what to expect—I had never seen anything like them. I felt intrigued: *This is going to be awesome!*

I leaned into my monitor, watching with anticipation, hanging on every word. Lainie pulled card after card, delivering the most delicious messages—I was instantly hooked! All the words and messages were spot on. In a Zoom room of many, I felt like the cards were talking directly to me. As she held the Cherries (Community) card, she spoke of her community of food healing; it sounded right up my alley. Another card that stood out was Pineapple (Expansion) Oh, yeah, I was, and also Lychee (Evolve). *Yes! It's time; I'm ready to know more and be more.*

Fireworks of ideas were going off in my mind. I wanted more.

Later that day, I signed up to become a Certified Intuitive Food Therapist. The classes took my experience to a whole new level. We learned about each card, its healing properties, the chakras, and the elements that went with each one. The possibilities were endless.

I started a daily game, asking myself: *What will the cards say today?*

I'd pull out the deck and start doing single-card draws, asking, *what is the energy around this day?* Or *What do I need to nourish my mind and body?*

As I continued the daily card pulls, I developed my intuition further—trusting whatever thought comes into my mind has a purpose. I felt better than ever—eating with pleasure and purpose. Not only did I release mental weight, but my waistline continued to decrease. I ate to *nourish* and less to punish or distract.

I no longer felt like I was at the mercy of my fork.

On Saturday mornings, before going to the grocery store, I pull a bunch of cards, lay them all out, and admire the beautiful pictures. Then, I use those cards to generate recipe ideas for the week.

Whether they're used in dishes or added to smoothies, while I eat them, I sit with each card, studying every detail of its beauty and reading each corresponding message, savoring what it means.

I became aware of why I was craving certain foods. I even learned about foods I never heard of in a new and exciting way.

The fridge was no longer my foe; it was my friend. I started seeing foods with new names. I chose a smoothie of love (strawberry), joy (mango), and clarity (blueberry) and drank it with mindfulness, intending to bring more of those feelings into my day. I wasn't only physically consuming food. I fed my mind at the same time. I felt satisfied and fulfilled with each meal.

A few months later, Lainie asked, "Would you like to do Oracle card readings at an in-person event?" I was nervous and scared. I had no idea the what or the how of it, but I knew the cards would deliver. My excitement to share nourishing messages and to try something new was much more significant than any fears trying to arise. Faith over fear and leading with *yes* became my motto for 2023 after all the lessons in 2022. So, I said, "Yes!"

I did several readings that day, but one will always sit in my heart. To respect privacy (and this story), we'll call her Emily.

Emily walked up to the booth where our readers were that day. Her mom chose one of the other ladies, and Emily picked me. Emily had never had a reading. She had never been to an event like that before. They happened to be staying at the nearby hotel, saw the event, and decided to check it out. We walked over to my table and introduced ourselves. I told her a bit about the cards and said a prayer: "Thank you, Spirit, for the gift of being able to do these readings today. I only allow 100% love and light to come into my space. Please remove my ego and only allow messages for their highest good to come through to me. Thank you, thank you, thank you."

I asked her, "Is there anything specific sitting on your heart or mind you'd like messages about?"

"Nothing, really," she said.

"Let's use our EMPS spread, which allows us to ask what the overall message for you today is regarding the emotional, mental, physical, and spiritual aspects."

"Sure, that sounds good."

As I pulled each card and set them facedown, I repeated in my mind:

Please allow this message to be clear and for me to interpret and communicate the message to give her the nourishment she needs.

Excitement and anticipation were building, both of us eager for what would come.

The first card, **Support**, the rich, orange butternut squash sliced in half, revealing a heart-shaped hole just waiting to support what needs to be held.

The second card, **Peace**, with two olives gently soaking together in the richness of the oil and filling the small white bowl.

The third, **Action**, bright, plump, juicy, ripe tomatoes ready to be plucked from the vine. There are also a few green ones that still need to be ready.

The final card, **Protection**, consists of several bulbs of garlic still encased in their papery layer, each clove ready to be revealed.

I saw her reaction to each card as they revealed: first, contemplation; then, we moved into the second, increased curiosity; then, with the third, a moment of realization started to happen; and with the final flip, awareness, and understanding as the message settled in and became clear.

What was so fascinating was that as I read through the book, I learned each card had medicinal properties for the heart. Emily then shared with me. "I had heart surgery many years ago and am in town for a getaway before heading back home to prepare for yet another surgery."

We sat there, looking at the cards, then at each other, and back to the cards. Both of us were in awe of the extraordinary message that unfolded.

The main takeaways of the EMPS reading were that emotionally, she had the support of her family. Mentally, it was peaceful knowing she had been through this before and had a good idea of what to expect. Physically, it was time to act, and the spiritual belief was that she wasn't alone (and protected in whatever would come).

I almost cried as she walked away, smiling, seemingly lighter and more at peace. What a special moment to share with what had been a total stranger. I truly felt the gift of our meeting not only for her but also for myself and the beautiful magic in these cards.

That moment was when I knew I wanted to share my newfound way of nourishing others with the world, and these messages were my new passion.

Whether you have a profound, burning question or are just looking for feedback from the universe, the cards always deliver, and the messages are spot on. It never gets old. I feel childlike excitement when they align just so.

Cards can be read in several different ways. Often, the message is about interpreting that word's meaning; sometimes, it's about the medicinal properties of the food, and other times, it's both.

In the beginning, intuitive, intentional eating takes practice; just like with anything, the more you do it over time, the more automatic it becomes. Answers to questions tend to resolve quicker and more clearly. Indecision and uncertainty subside. Knowing throughout the day that you are exactly where you're meant to be, doing what you are supposed to be doing sets in. The world becomes more peaceful and connected; overall, you feel more aligned.

Mealtime is no longer a source of pain, punishment, or guilt—it's fun, adventurous, and fulfilling.

THE TOOL

Use the foods in your kitchen and your intuition to receive tasty messages right at home.

There're several kinds of card spreads to satisfy any questions you may have. While the cards I mentioned in my story feature delicious, vibrant foods, I'll walk you through a reading without any cards at all.

Today, we'll use my favorite spread, the EMPS

(Emotional, Mental, Physical, and Spiritual).

PREPARATION

First, I highly recommend a pen and journal.

Second, take a moment to center or ground yourself. Take three deep breaths. Inhale for a count of three, hold for three, then exhale for three.

Third, set the intention with a gratitude prayer of your choice, "Thank you for the opportunity to connect with you today; please allow me to see, feel, and hear the messages needed for my best and highest good."

Last, speak your question aloud or in your mind, and be open and ready to receive. Example question for this exercise: *What's the energy and message for the day ahead?*

Step 1: Find the food to deliver the message.

Stand in the kitchen, take a moment just to be there, take in the room's energy, close your eyes, and take in the smells and the sounds. Notice your body. Do you feel it leaning in a particular direction? Open your eyes and move in that direction. Open the doors if you are in front of the fridge or pantry. Look for an item that seems brighter than the rest and appears to be calling to you. *This* is the tasty morsel I want to speak to you today.

Step 2: Connect

Hold the food in your hand, observe every inch, touch all the sides, bring it to your nose, and inhale the aromas. Speak to it, ask it your question, or give a simple hello. Be aware of how you are feeling and what thoughts are coming to your mind. Take as long in this moment as you feel is right.

Step 3: Receive the message.

As you are holding your food, let's go thru the EMPS

A tip for this step is to trust the first thoughts that come into your mind. Be sure to write these down; don't analyze them, just get them on paper. They'll come together in the end.

Emotional: What are you feeling inside? Joy, peace, acceptance, calm, envy, love. Do you want to cry or laugh? Are you being reminded of a prior time or event in your life?

Mental: How is your thinking? Clear or confused, tired or excited, take note of your attitude and what words are coming to your mind.

Physical: Notice your body. Are you noticing any sensations, tingling, or pressure? Is the body light or heavy, hot or cold? Is your heartbeat slow or fast? Are you feeling the urge to jump, run, or more called to be still and relaxed?

Spirit: Are thoughts nudging you to connect more often and deeper? Are the words medication or prayer coming up for you? Or are there ideas on ways to feel more aligned with Spirit?

Sit with the words you've written and give gratitude for the connection to the food and its message to your mind, body, and spirit. If you feel so inclined, nourish yourself with the tasty morsel that delivered its messages to you while you reflect.

Our foods have so many tasty messages ready to deliver to us. All we must do is ask, connect, and receive.

The cards amplify the message and deepen the connection. Let's connect to see what nourishing messages the cards hold for you.

SAMPLE READING

"What is the energy and message for this chapter contribution?"

EMOTIONAL—MEDITATION/FIGS

Several figs adorn the card. One cut in half looks like an amethyst geode, with its internal purple goodness glistening. Another is upright, with its green stem pointing up to the sky.

Meditation is not a dirty word. It doesn't have to involve sitting still for long periods and trying to control your thoughts; it can be as simple as just a few minutes doing anything that brings quiet to your mind.

Message: To get to the right mindset, spend time in the quiet. Prepare with sound healing, guided meditation, and teatime while basking in Mother Nature. Quiet your mind from the busyness and allow yourself to open your mind, body, and spirit to hear the message to share today.

The element is spirit, connecting to your higher self to bring forward nourishing messages.

The chakra is the crown; we seek knowledge, understanding, and fulfillment.

MENTAL—LEMONS/ALCHEMY

A bright yellow, fresh-cut lemon sits atop a white hand juicer, just waiting for the yummy juice to be squeezed into existence.

Wow! So, this is so cool. When I first embarked on this endeavor, the alchemy card kept coming up.

Message: I wasn't sure how to write a chapter or what message to share, but I trusted Spirit to guide the way, and if my heart and integrity were aligned, the message to be shared would flow. Part of spiritual alchemy is freedom from our fears and the release of parts of ourselves that are ready to be changed and evolved. Again, the spirit element and crown chakra are represented here. Coincidence? I think not.

PHYSICAL—COFFEE/ENERGY

I can smell the coffee as I look at the cluster of beans. Some reflect light, and others have a dark, shadowy mystery.

Message, I hear; *what energy do you hope to convey to the world with your message?* I want to help others experience freedom from the fork and have beautiful gifts of joy, peace, and overall wellness.

This card has several elements: earth, air, fire, and the chakra is the root.

SPIRITUAL—OLIVES/PEACE

Several green olives are placed in different ways. A small white bowl filled with oil holds two shiny olives soaking together in its richness. Even more are spread over the table, waiting for their turn to bask in the goodness.

Message: When the story is shared and the message is delivered, I hope to have given a gift: Peace of mind and within the heart.

This card has two elements: earth and air, and the chakra is the crown.

I hope you enjoyed that morsel of fun and learned to love mealtime again.

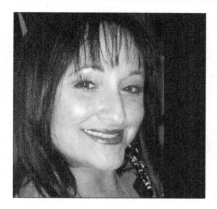

Kari Bozic is a mom, wife, daughter, sister, and friend to many. She's a Florida-born native who's had the opportunity to travel all over the US but calls Southwest Florida home.

Kari struggled with mental and physical health issues for decades until awakening to intuitive, intentional eating in 2022.

She's a Certified level 1 and 2 Intuitive Food Therapist who enjoys providing nourishing, intuitive messages for the mind, body, and spirit using the *Food Healing Oracle Deck*®.

Kari strives to bring love, peace, and healing to others by introducing them to a new way of looking at food, showing them how to use intention and intuition with each meal to lead a more balanced life. She'll teach you to stop eating to deflect, self-medicate, or sabotage and start nourishing for the best and highest good.

She's had the opportunity to have the right people placed on her path at the right time to be the light needed, and now she wants to be that light for others. She believes when you illuminate the world, how can it not shine back on you?

Kari's a woman living an elevated, enlightened life. It all started with loving and accepting herself completely and unconditionally, and it opened the gates for her to trust herself and live a life of faith and flow.

Do you want to learn to eat to nourish and not to punish? She'll show you how in a fun, exciting way.

As the Food Healing Oracle Deck® says, "You will never look at food the same again."

Kari invites you to reach. "Let's play with our food together."

Konnect with Kari:

Facebook: www.facebook.com/KariKonnects
Instagram: Kari_Konnects(@karikonnects)
Website: https://karikonnects.com

CHAPTER 5

THE RAINDROP TECHNIQUE

UNLOCKING ESSENTIAL OIL SECRETS FOR TOTAL MIND-BODY RELAXATION

Ruth S. Bailey, CRTS, LSH, MSW

MY STORY

You're always one decision away from a totally different life; it's essential to choose wisely.

At the beginning of the pandemic, I felt a strong urge to step off the beaten path of my career. *I can't continue to go into a work environment that doesn't bring me joy; this is depleting my happiness. I must make a change.* Trusting my instincts and pivoting to a new career was like choosing to go in the opposite direction of traffic, but it was the best decision I ever made. Even though it can be daunting to take the road less traveled in a world where career paths are often predefined, sometimes following our calling and pursuing what truly ignites our spirit is the way to go. If you're at a crossroads in your life, remember that there is always time for a thrilling plot twist in your story.

What is it that keeps you up at night?

I was constantly being distracted by my thoughts at work. I clocked in and sat down to begin my day, and the daydreaming started. Ever been in love? It's similar to when you're passionate about embarking on a new chapter in your career. Your thoughts are continually on that person, and at times, you find yourself smiling when thinking about them. The love of my life, this new love I found, is helping and educating others about health and wellness. I shared my dreams of changing career tracks with close family and friends. When you share your passion, magic happens.

Ruth: Hello Beautiful, I've been meaning to bring you an update with my changes to my career.

Close Friend: I would love to hear, I'm all ears.

Ruth: My love for essential oils is no secret. I've found a technique that combines oils and therapeutic touch. It's called the Raindrop Technique. Have you heard of it?

Close Friend: Yes, that moment when stress left my body, and serenity took its place. I didn't want to get off the table, girl. Talk about total mind-body relaxation. I love how it's a whole-body connection. Have you thought about Raindrop for pets? Or possibly traveling to facilitate Raindrop sessions? I know of someone knowledgeable in that area. I can get you in contact with them.

Ruth: I would very much appreciate that connection. You're continually helping me expand my thoughts. I will look into Raindrop for pets. Yes, traveling to facilitate Raindrop sessions is already something I'm doing; I'm looking forward to having more frequent opportunities.

I experienced this magnificent magic on several occasions. I shared what I was looking forward to accomplishing and a friend connected me to someone knowledgeable in the area. It's essential to have a trusting relationship with friends you can reflect with and bounce ideas off of. I see trust as the first step toward healing and stress relief. Building trust opens doors to wellness and fosters joy.

You are planning to do what? I'm planning to leave my nine-to-five job after 20 years with the organization. *Why?* Ever stared fear in the face and said, "Not today!?" Overcoming fear isn't about having no fear; it's about dancing with it and facing it head-on. On this journey of changing career paths and moving from corporate to entrepreneurship, internal thoughts kept me stuck. *How am I going to afford my own health insurance? Am I capable of going against the norm? How am I going to handle bills without a consistent biweekly income?*

I also realized I needed to be careful about what I shared with family who asked questions that stirred up fear. I faced each fear head-on. For health insurance, a close friend connected me to an agent who was able to assist me. Navigating internal conflict is a vital skill. Learning to mediate our inner disputes can lead to enhanced decision-making and better stress management. I continue to work on my internal conflict through self-development, working with mentors, and listening to motivational podcasts and videos. I learned to leverage my apprehension as a stepping stone. I was born to live my dream, not my fear.

Have you ever felt deep down inside your bones that you're designed for more? Do you ever wake up feeling like there's more to your professional journey? I've learned that feeling is more than intuition; it's a call to action. At this point in my life, I'm willing to take that risk and pursue my dreams of reinventing myself. Growth is synonymous with stepping out of one's comfort zone. The truth? Real change and innovation never sprouted from being comfortable.

I'd like to pause to express my deep gratitude for a remarkable woman who left an indelible mark on my life. My mother, an extraordinary force of nature, not only taught me the power of resilience, dedication, and compassion but embodied these qualities every day. With her unwavering strength and boundless empathy, my mother has been the guiding light illuminating my path toward a career centered on social work and wellness. Who was that person in your life?

A simple encounter with my mom propelled me to the next level of pursuing my passion. One day, I accompanied her to a doctor's visit; during the time at the office, the doctor diagnosed her with thyroid issues. The suggestion was made to remove her thyroid. I observed my mother as she sat still for a short instant, then began to make her face into some expression of 'I don't think so.' She looked at the doctor and said, "I don't want to do surgery. What are some natural ways to support my body?" At this moment, I decided to help my mother find a holistic option instead of removing her thyroid and relying on medication for the rest of her life. She wanted to explore natural alternatives.

Reflecting on my childhood, I'm flooded with fond memories of how my mother always turned to natural remedies to nurse me back to health whenever my adventurous spirit led to inevitable mishaps. Each recollection brings a warm smile, especially when I reminisce about the exhilarating moments of climbing trees. While ascending was always exciting, the descent often presented a thrilling challenge that tested my courage and agility.

Next I'll share about one of the most powerful natural remedies I've used to help me move through life and bust through the fears. I've discovered the subtle yet profound impact of essential oils on wellness and emotional resilience.

THE TOOL

During the pandemic, isolation and no contact were enforced. In these times, the power of touch was our silent hero. I've seen first-hand how therapeutic touch can transform our well-being. It's more than a feel-good moment; it's about connection, healing, and reminding us that we're not alone. Realizing the importance and benefits of touch, especially during the pandemic, made me even more passionate about facilitating the Raindrop Technique. A simple touch can boost our immune system, lower stress levels, and brighten our days. Touch is a universal language that communicates, "I'm here for you." Touch is a superpower we all have.

My journey into the world of essential oils was no accident. From day one, smelling the essential oils and being able to shift my mood—I knew I was onto something special—God's natural remedies in the small bottles. That's why I've been captivated by the healing power of essential oils and drawn to the Raindrop Technique. It's a powerful combination of essential oils and touch. I've dived head-first into this because, let's face it, traditional health solutions aren't always the answer. Many people are on a quest for alternative health solutions. This method isn't just about relaxation; it's a transformative process that enhances well-being, aiming to bridge the gap between traditional and alternative health practices. Witnessing the transformation firsthand brings me so much joy, and making the change in my career was so worth it. Let's redefine wellness standards.

We live in a society where symptoms are being treated, not the root cause. We can see the impact on our mental state and bodies from harboring deep resentment, as well as the benefits of releasing and forgiving, which can be healing. For us to become whole and healthy effectively, we must balance the mind, body, and spirit. Sometimes, we may feel under the weather, and the root cause isn't what you'd expect. There is a strong connection between illness and deep-rooted resentment. In the realm of health and wellness, understanding the psychological underpinnings of illness is crucial. I see time and time again how releasing resentment leads to amazing health improvements. It's time to detox those emotions, not only your body. Let's raise our high vibrational wellness by forgiving, forgetting, and flourishing.

The Raindrop Technique was developed by the late D. Gary Young, who first chose the nine pure therapeutic grade essential oils for specific reasons such as to kill viral and bacterial pathogens, support the immune system, reduce inflammation, ease respiratory discomfort, relieve the body of bone and joint discomfort, and relax stressed muscles. He accumulated from his experience with Native American wellness traditions and delivered a revolutionary means of aligning the body and mind.

This unique technique has the facilitator start at the feet and move up the spine using a roll-and-release method, targeting several key reflex areas along the way. The Raindrop Technique involves dropping essential oils along the spine and using light feather strokes to move the oil into the skin. The Raindrop Technique also includes Vita-Flex on the bottom of the feet and ends with a warm compress on the back. A powerful, relaxing treatment that offers several benefits to the mind, body, and spirit. Raindrop Technique is an experience for everyone at any age for whatever their need or desire may be. It has also been used on pets. Below are the essential oils used in the Raindrop Technique:

1. Oregano: Powerful immune stimulant, anti-fungal, anti-inflammatory.

2. Thyme: One of the most powerful anti-bacterial essential oils, anti-parasitic, anti-microbial. Helps to overcome fatigue and exhaustion after illness.

3. Basil: Anti-spasmodic, anti-inflammatory, anti-bacterial, relaxant, fights mental fatigue, and releases muscle tension.

4. Wintergreen: Supports the respiratory tract, pain relief for arthritis, joints, muscles and nerves, anti-spasmodic.

5. Cypress: Improves circulation, strengthens blood capillaries.

6. Peppermint: Digestive stimulant, cooling oil, anti-inflammatory, anti-viral, anti-bacterial.

7. Marjoram: Known as the herb of happiness, calms the nerves, has muscle-soothing properties, general relaxant.

8. Valor oil blend: Structural balancing and alignment, gives a boost to confidence and self-esteem, balances electrical energies in the body.

9. Aroma Siez oil blend: An exclusive blend of basil, marjoram, lavender, peppermint, and cypress that has an invigorating yet calming aroma and produces soothing comfort for fatigued muscles.

Gary wanted to empower everyone in their wellness journey, so an at-home experience fits perfectly with that vision. Below are instructions on how to apply the essential oils to your own feet.

STEP 1: PREPARATION

Provide a calming environment. Create a relaxing setting with a comfortable temperature, no noises or distractions, and dimmed lighting. Having short-trimmed fingernails is required. You'll need these oils and blends in the order of: Valor, oregano, thyme, basil, cypress, wintergreen, marjoram, Aroma Size, peppermint, and White Angelica. White Angelica is not part of the collection, but its frequency neutralizes negative energy and gives a feeling of security.

STEP 2: APPLY VALOR ESSENTIAL OIL BLEND

Drop three to six drops of Valor blend in the palm of your right hand and rub it on the bottom of your left foot. Next, drop three to six drops of Valor blend in the palm of your left hand and rub it on the bottom of your right foot. Place the palm of your right hand on the bottom of your left foot. Place the palm of your left hand on the bottom of your right foot. Hold this position for three to five minutes.

STEP 3: ROLL AND RELEASE

Place two to three drops of oregano oil into your left palm, then circle the fingertips of your right hand around your left palm three times clockwise. Place your right hand on the spinal reflex point at the heel. The spinal reflex point is located from the top of your hallux/great toe to your heel. Roll your fingers slowly until your nails are flat against the bottom of your foot, then back to the original position, starting at your heel. Repeat along the entire length of the foot's spinal reflex points and off the great toe, moving up one-quarter of an inch each time, repeating three times.

Place two to three drops of oregano oil into your right palm, then circle the fingertips of your left hand around your right palm three times clockwise. Place your left hand on the spinal reflex point at the heel. Roll your fingers slowly until your nails are flat against the bottom of your foot, then back to the original position. Repeat along the entire length of the foot's spinal reflex points and off the great toe, moving up one-quarter of an inch each time, repeating three times.

Apply the roll and release technique on the right foot using the left hand and the left foot using the right hand. Repeat the roll release technique with thyme, basil, cypress, wintergreen, marjoram, and peppermint in the order listed.

In my latest encounter with the transformative powers of the Raindrop Technique, a client reported significant improvement in mobility, pain reduction, and better sleep quality. A few days later, I called to follow up, and the client reported that they could sleep in their bed instead of using the recliner. Previous to a Raindrop session, many nights were spent in the recliner because sleeping in bed was too painful. This case underscores not only the potential of alternative wellness practices in enhancing quality of life but also the gratification of facilitating these breakthroughs. I'm driven by the belief that we can redefine well-being, one drop at a time.

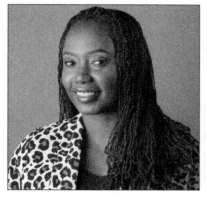

Ruth S. Bailey is a Certified Raindrop Technique Specialist, social worker, licensed spiritual healer, and health and wellness coach. Throughout her career, Ruth continues to study in areas to add to her knowledge such as aromatherapy and the aroma freedom technique. Her business is called Holistic Journey. Ruth found a fantastic location to facilitate her Raindrop Technique sessions. This space aligns perfectly with her vision of promoting health and well-being in a tranquil environment.

Ruth Bailey was born in Guyana, South America, she moved to the United States in 1992 and currently resides in Upstate New York. Her parents wanted a better education for her and her two sisters. Migrating for education represents more than just an academic pursuit; it's a transformative journey fostering unparalleled growth, both personally and professionally.

Ruth enjoys spending time with family and friends, traveling, educating about essential oils, and being a positive light that radiates love. She believes the leaves of the trees are nature's very own remedy cabinet, designed by the ultimate healer—God. Ruth is inspired to share a natural healing method to help women remove excess stressors and toxicity from their lives.

Connecting with Ruth all begins with a 30-minute complimentary discovery chat to discuss your wellness needs and vision and discover how Ruth can best support you on this journey towards better health. Allow Ruth to journey with you to provide accountability and guidance.

Connect with Ruth:

Facebook: https://www.facebook.com/ruth.love.73/

Email: info@journeywithruth.com

LinkTree Link: https://linktr.ee/ruthbailey28

CHAPTER 6

CONNECTING TO THE POWER OF THE HIGHER CONSCIOUSNESS

CREATING INNER PEACE AFTER EMOTIONALLY ABUSIVE RELATIONSHIPS

Cheryle Freedman, LCSW, PsyD

"You've always had the power, my dear,
you just had to learn it for yourself."

~ Glinda, the Good Witch, The Wizard of Oz, Frank L. Baum

MY STORY

After a series of emotionally abusive relationships, I was mentally and physically exhausted.

As a child, I spent eight years living with a narcissistic mother and an abusive stepfather, distressing enough that I don't even remember parts of my childhood. Then, on to a narcissistic husband who believed all the things wrong in his life were my fault and told me so every day. The deep aching pain in my heart finally erupted into uncontrollable sobbing as I wondered: *Is it even worth it? Maybe I shouldn't be here. No one will even miss me.* But something inside me had other ideas.

Don't you give up! Your work here isn't done. You're needed!

Where did that come from? Now, I'm hearing voices.

I didn't realize I'd just made first contact with the power within me.

I later discovered that its name was the Higher Consciousness (HC). Eventually, my "yellow brick road" brought me to the energy healing techniques of past life regression and Beyond Quantum Healing. The HC and I are now on a first-name basis, and I always ask for its help. This vibrational healing nourished my mind, body, and spirit despite years of abusive relationships and brought me the inner peace I never knew. And I'm here to help others find the power to create that peace within themselves.

Higher consciousness is a state of awareness that is your direct connection between source energy and the information written on your soul, known as your divine blueprint. This blueprint holds all the wisdom you've gathered throughout time, space, and dimension, from your ancient past to a future you have yet to live. The HC is the path to discovering your inner power for healing. However, you must ask for help as it believes in free will and won't intervene without your permission.

At thirty-eight, my husband of nineteen years walks out the door.

"I need to leave." Paralyzed, no words spill from my mouth. My stomach tightened as my 14-year-old son, 17-year-old daughter, and I watched in frozen silence as he left.

"Is he coming back?" my son said.

"I don't know."

What can I tell them? Maybe it's a mistake. He's been so distant for the past year, but I didn't expect this! Don't let them see how scared you are. Hold it together, Cheryle.

Tears threatened to spill, but I didn't want to upset my kids. "It's going to be okay." But it isn't. We go about our daily routines, kids going to school and me going to work, pretending everything is fine. I never tell any of my coworkers. A week goes by before I even hear from him, and then he refuses to tell me where he is or how to get in touch with him. I eventually learn he's living with the girl he's been seeing for the past year, the year I've been recovering from cancer.

Food makes me gag, so I live on cigarettes and Diet Pepsi. I lost 14 pounds in two weeks, dropping my weight to 105 pounds, and I can't sleep without wine to knock me out. Still, I awaken at 2 a.m. every night, negative thoughts swirling through my mind. Abusive relationships left me with countless negative feelings about myself. You know the ones I'm talking about, the kinds that poison your mind with mean and ugly lies about your self-worth and steal your peace and happiness. I wanted to believe I deserved better, but I took up where he left off and continued to berate myself with the same poisonous words.

The mind, body, and spirit are so interconnected that lower vibrational thoughts such as "it's my fault, I'm worthless, I'm ashamed" may lead to feelings of fear, anger, and stress, impacting physical well-being. That's what happened to me. These thoughts poisoned my mind and made me sick! My health deteriorated due to these lower vibrational limiting beliefs. To restore balance, I had to nourish my mind with high-vibrational thoughts like gratitude for the lessons I learned, the skills I developed (I repaired the sheetrock he put his fist through), and knowing I had the love of my two children to guide me through the hard times. So, I nourished my mind with thoughts that heal, not harm. You can, too.

Five years after my divorce, I finally moved on. But peace and happiness still eluded me. Then, I woke up and realized the fairy tale knight wouldn't ride up on his white horse and save me.

I need to make myself happy. I think I'll go camping next weekend. It'll feel good to hang out in nature and read a book. Maybe I'll see if I can volunteer for the ambulance on my days off from the hospital. You know, it feels pretty good that I can go where I want when I want without having to ask permission! I might even get my hair highlighted.

Then, a nice guy from work asked me out, and we started dating. I met his parents two months later, and the old insecurities surfaced.

What if they hate me? After all, I'm eight years older than him, divorced, have adult children, and only have an associate degree in nursing. He's a doctor, for crying out loud! They won't think I'm good enough for him. Hell, I don't think I'm good enough! I'm going to be sick.

Too late. The door opens, and a petite woman with gray hair floating around her face envelops my boyfriend in her arms.

"Come in, come in! Say hi to Dad!"

"Mom, Dad, this is Cheryle."

They engulf us in big hugs and smiles, and my heartbeat slows to a normal rhythm.

"Please call us Tee and David. Cheryle, we'll go sit in the living room and get to know each other while Eric talks with Dad."

"Eric said you have a private practice, Tee. What is it you do?"

"Hypnosis and past life regression."

Eyes wide, I sit forward in my chair.

"I use it as a healing modality. Recently, I saw a woman who had tried several times to take her children to see the battlefield at Gettysburg, but the minute she stepped out of the car, she started crying and couldn't walk onto the field. In hypnosis, she reported being the mother of a soldier who died at Gettysburg and was buried there. But he was from Virginia. Her past life personality made a promise to bring his body back to Virginia for burial, but she passed without fulfilling the promise. I asked her to picture her past life self, standing before the son, telling him she was sorry she couldn't keep her promise. She was then able to release the guilt. After that, in her current life, she could go view Gettysburg without a problem!"

"But how did she do that? How was she able to release the guilt?"

"With the help of the Higher Consciousness."

This was the first time I heard the name Higher Consciousness, and I thought: *This might be what I've been looking for! If the Higher Consciousness can heal, I want to know how to connect!*

I began training with Tee soon after, and as they say, the rest is history. As a side note, Eric and I married two years later. It'll be thirty years this July!

Telling my story brings back some pain, but I'm doing it to let you know that, just like me (and Dorothy,) you too have the power to rebuild your self-worth and find your inner peace, regardless of the fire you've walked through. You deserve to have a life filled with peace and happiness.

Glinda was right. I had to learn it for myself.

You'll need to "learn it for yourself," too. But you're not alone. The HC and I will help you find your power.

THE TOOL

A few years ago, I created Spiritual Stargates, which are best described as metaphorical portals designed to take you from where you are currently in life to the transformation you desire to see. To pass through a stargate, you must match the vibrational energy of each unique portal. Spiritual Stargates are the energy techniques I use to help clients connect their Higher Consciousness to all the wisdom they hold within their divine blueprint but have no access to on a conscious level. This hidden information holds what you need to create the changes you desire.

Higher consciousness is an elevated state of awareness that operates at the high end of the vibrational energy scale. Uplifting thoughts such as gratitude, love, and empowerment are a vibrational match for connection with the power of the HC and allow you to pass through the portal. Thoughts like guilt, shame, or jealousy are lower on the vibrational scale and, therefore, not a match for connecting with the Higher Consciousness.

The power of the HC lies in helping you access the information you have deep within and in helping you zoom out to a level where you can see the bigger picture and change your perspective about a situation or person. Changes you make via the Higher Consciousness come about because you're guided to consider things you didn't see when you were stuck in a conflict. Tapping into this elevated state of being provides the opportunity for profound personal growth, increased clarity, and a deeper connection to the world and people around you. Changing your perspective can change your feelings about a negative situation and enable you to see something you may have now that you wouldn't have had if the situation had not forced a change.

Beyond Quantum Healing is the main (Spiritual Stargate) tool I use. The client and I speak directly with the Higher Consciousness, asking questions the client wants answered, such as "Am I following the right path? Should I make a change in my job?" Additionally, we ask for the HC's help in healing any issues with mind, body, or spirit, even those the client may not be aware of. I often ask the HC to describe the healing process as it works, and it tells me that it's using "white light energy."

This interaction occurs during a hypnosis-based session and *must be facilitated by a trained practitioner.* However, there are Spiritual Stargates you can use on your own to connect with the Higher Consciousness and request its help. I'm including two here to get you started.

GUIDED VISUALIZATION PRACTICE

This can be done at bedtime or during the day. It works best with your eyes closed, so either memorize the script or record yourself on your phone to playback.

- Lie in a comfortable place where you will not be disturbed (or when you lie down in bed).

- Play relaxing background music (if needed) without words or singing.

- Say: "I ask my angels, spirit guides, ascended masters, and source energy to help me in this process; I ask that only the most benevolent beings who serve my highest and best interest come forward." Then say or think the following:

- "Higher Consciousness, I need your help with the following problem or healing (Insert what you are asking for here.) I'm not sure how to do this myself, so I'm asking for your help. Please work on this as I sleep (or after my daily practice) and send me the answer in any way you deem appropriate. Help me to be aware of the message.

Note: The Higher Consciousness will send you the message at a time it feels is appropriate. I have awakened some mornings with the answer to a tech problem I was having difficulty with, so you can see, it's not just for emotional, physical, and spiritual healing! Just keep asking.

MEDITATION FOR CREATING INNER PEACE

Again, sit in a comfortable place where you won't be disturbed, and gently close your eyes. You can either record yourself or click below to join my email list and receive the link to download my free audio recording, which includes background music.

Sit back, relax, and gently close your eyes as we focus on peace, the ultimate vibration that will guide us to fulfill our Divine Blueprint.

There is no greater gift we can give the planet or ourselves, especially during these trying times.

We are physically living these lessons; lessons we agreed to learn, knowing that we chose to be here in this time and space to assist humanity in recognizing that many must become one.

Now, begin to focus within,

to your core being,

your Original Source Energy.

It is here that great changes can be made.

Your source energy is your soul energy.

And your soul energy understands that you cannot create peace in the world until you can create peace within yourself.

That is the first step.

Begin by practicing gratitude.

Each day, notice all that you have to be grateful for.

Focus on forgiving those who have hurt you, understanding that forgiveness does not mean you are okay with what others have done.

It means you are releasing that negative energy, the hurt, and anger that remains within you,

so that you create inner peace.

You cannot change another person; you can only change yourself.

But when you change yourself,

when you become one with peace,

when you replace the hurt and anger with unconditional love, it affects those around you, and that is what will produce the change.

We are vibrational beings, emitting waves of energy out into the world,

and others feel that energy.

They take it in, and they begin to feel unconditional love.

At this time in history, when peace in the world is often so elusive,

begin by creating peace within yourself.

That peace will spread to those around you,

out to the world, out to the Universe and beyond.

When that vibrational energy reaches the spiritual planes, our guides will send it back to us, completing the circle that will bring peace and love to the world.

Allow that love to be within you every day.

Take this gentle, loving feeling with you as you leave here today,

and allow it to remain within you always.

As you shine your inner light, peace and love will spread throughout all dimensions, and that love will heal the planet. And so, it is.

You may open your eyes when ready, feeling relaxed and refreshed.

*Receive a bonus audio of this meditation (with background music) when you sign up for my email list. http://eepurl.com/iMXC3c

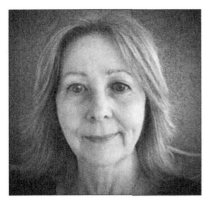

Dr. Cheryle Freedman is originally from Upstate New York but now lives with her husband, Eric, in Cape Coral, Florida. She is a Licensed Clinical Social Worker, Doctor of Psychology, with a Concentration in Hypnotherapy and Counseling, and certified Beyond Quantum Healing Practitioner (BQH) who helps clients make transformational changes by connecting with their past lives and the Higher Consciousness. She's also an Advanced Theta Healing Practitioner and certified Food Healing Oracle Deck® reader. She employs these and other holistic practices to complement her BQH sessions.

Cheryle worked as an emergency department registered nurse for 15 years before earning her MSSW from Rockefeller College in Albany, New York. As a psychotherapist, she conducted trauma therapy with sexually abused children for 12 years and testified on their behalf in family court. Her doctoral studies focused on trauma and memory.

She has used past life regression with her clients for 30 years, specifically as a healing modality, and is passionate about helping her clients release physical, emotional, and spiritual pain without causing further trauma. The insight gained in past life reviews often leads to healing in the current life.

Cheryle became more immersed in holistic practices in Florida, eventually joining the local Holistic Chamber of Commerce, where she met and learned from other holistic providers.

Cheryle is the author of *Raven Can't Sleep*, a guided imagery children's book and accompanying CD for children with worries and sleep challenges. She is a spiritual recording artist with tracks on several Gulf Coast Meditations CDs, including Abundance, Children, Tweens & Teens, and Sleep, and an individual CD: The Keys, Vol. III, Meditations & Messages for Life's Most Challenging Times.

To learn more about Cheryle and BQH:

Website: https://spiritualstargates.com

Facebook: https://www.facebook.com/PastLifeArcheologist

Contact: cheryle@spiritualstargates.com

CHAPTER 7

CRAVINGS

WHAT YOUR BODY IS TELLING YOU AND WHAT TO DO ABOUT IT

Linda McBee, Publisher

MY STORY

That roller coaster ride never seems to stop.

I'm more than sixty pounds overweight. Food and sugar were how I dealt with the stress of losing my mom after six months of cancer. Dad sold the farmhouse, and with it went the big stream running through the property and the massive garden covering the recently purchased backyard. Some of my fondest pictures are still vibrant in my memory of Mom cooking everything from scratch. It still brings a warm, cozy energy to me.

Food was an important connection I was taught as a child from the smell and taste of a great home-cooked meal and an emotion I still feel today. Little did I know how quickly it would turn from being positive to negative.

Nana, Dad's mother, whom I lived with for about a year, was 4'11" and 97 pounds. She ran a restaurant for most of her life and served well-balanced meals. The emotional love I received from her helped start a new chapter in my life as a five-year-old navigating the world with no mother.

I remember Nana's smile as she poured me a small cup of half milk and half coffee stirred tenderly with a little sugar. She was making toast for dunking (as a treat). My coffee cravings are the emotional love from my Nana. I knew she put her heart in my special drink—it put a huge smile on my face. I was encouraged to play with the neighbor girls down by the stream or at their home so I could have those special recollections of being a kid. These would be cherished memories that I'd long for.

Riding on the wheel well with my hair blowing in the breeze as we went to the barn to feed the horses with Papaw was another highlight of the day. I also rode bareback—I grabbed the mane and held on for dear life. My horse led the pack to the stream in the woods while I laughed at the top of my lungs from the thrill. This created some normalcy in my not-so-normal life. My family was traumatized, as was I. Mom arranged that after her passing, we would stay with Nana and Papaw.

Grandma, Mom's mother, was German and a widow herself from the time my mom was a little girl and was now dealing with the loss of her daughter. The memories with Grandma flooded in, like having my cousins visit, walking to K-Mart, walking around the blocks in Gettysburg, smelling kielbasa cooking (my wakeup call), and having small amounts of Kahlua on the rocks. My fatty cravings were wonderful memories of my grandma, and the Kahlua made for a wonderful dessert. I can't remember when this tradition started but having a shot glass with ice and a splash of yumminess (which we sipped on for hours) were fond memories.

As the year passed, my family cried with the abrupt death and deep loss we experienced. I was mortified trying to comprehend life. "What are you doing today, Mom?" I asked with swollen eyes as I looked at the sky. "Are you visiting with Grandpa, who passed when you were a little girl? What is heaven like? I'd love to watch you cook and experience the joy you had as you sang and the happy energy you exuded while you created art we thoroughly enjoyed." This visual is only in my memories now. Instead, I find myself crying on the inside with a poker face and miles away, lost in confusion without any words. Emotional eating became a true reality. Anything sweet was my go-to, and I hit it hard, revolving into an emotional eater to hide the pain. I hurt and didn't know where to turn, so sugar got my full attention.

Dad processed his sadness by finding a "mom." He now lived farther away from work; the highlight was receiving a kiss when he got home. "Does anyone have a sister who's single," he asked his class. He was introduced to Ann, whom he married eight months later. "Take your time," Nana said. "Don't rush into anything." "I just want to get back to normal," he said. "Linda, you should come live with us."

Ann's therapist suggested she shouldn't marry. They didn't listen, and now being abused was part of my daily routine. My happy-go-lucky temperament created a jealous rage, resulting in her grabbing my arms, and as her voice got louder, her grip stronger, and often red marks lingered. Saying she was hurting me or showing any emotion resulted in additional episodes. Poker face generated fewer tirades but caused increased sleepless nights, crying in my pillow with nowhere to turn.

One of the other devastating memories, often ignored, was when I asked for a drink (since I couldn't reach a cup). I learned quickly that the bathroom and my hands could supply hydration. This taught me resourcefulness, which was very important later in life. Lack of care was common, with the cupboards and refrigerator bare and very limited food available. Every plate from the cupboard was dirty and stacked up sky-high, and there was no space available to do anything in the kitchen. My environment was a hoarder's house with stacks of papers everywhere. I created reasons to have sleepovers and time with neighbors' kids to avoid the abandonment I felt.

My worst nightmare happened again with Ann. It was my next birthday when I had friends and family over. In the middle of playing games outside, she appeared disheveled, screaming and crying, "I shouldn't have married; this marriage is horrible, and I should get a divorce." I was mortified. My birthday is in the summer, and I was upset when the kids brought it up the next time I saw them at school. That was the last time I asked for a party growing up.

Sneaking extra food became a game since the cravings were intense. Continuing to get heavier and struggling with body image created a roller coaster ride that was on replay. Being overweight was playing havoc on my self-image. *I want to be a part of that softball team that always wins. I want to be invited to that party with all the skinny girls.* I wanted to be picked first on the dodgeball team, but I was picked last.

In my early teens, I was introduced to a doctor that was all about health and wellness. This gave me the energy and nutrition my body needed to feel better about myself because I started paying attention to the food I ate and stayed away from so much sugar. His education about sugar and how it can cause addictions challenged me to find better, more nutritious solutions for my sweet cravings. Cooking opened the door to experimenting with foods and spices, focusing on how I felt when I ate. My mom inspired and taught me to love to cook, and I feel she's still supporting me on this journey. I'm thankful she's orchestrated all the angels to help me heal my inner child and be who I am today. These lessons taught me to work through my emotional, mental, spiritual, and physical cravings—I eat to live instead of live to eat.

Puzzling as it might be, Ann was very supportive in my health journey. She created snacks and things that helped change my eating habits for a lifetime. She was very skinny and loved to control situations (realizing this was something she could control for me), and she did. It helped give me the discipline that has carried me through my life. The program was on counting calories, but I focused on eating more vegetables, fruits, and protein and getting away from processed foods and sugary condiments.

Tenacity gave me the discipline in life to complete high school. Working on my cravings and addictions while receiving a mental health therapy degree was a monumental milestone, and I was incredibly proud of myself. Pursuing training in food, health, and human interaction was critical in my healing. Becoming a functional medicine coach helped me see how my past blood reports and blood type were affected by the foods I ate. I gave up gluten and focused on foods that were more acceptable according to my blood type, and it's been a massive game-changer. A Human Interaction Techniques certification taught me to change the images in my mind from negative, sad pictures to positive, happy ones by using activities to work through the trauma. PTSD caused me to bury the gory details of my past. Thankfully, with this training, I learned to create different, transformational images, helping me to show up differently to myself and others. Before the class, the intense PTSD caused me to focus only on how distressing life was with Ann, not the good from her nor any experiences from my mom. The Human Interaction Technique assisted me in resolving Ann's actions that didn't serve me. I needed to forgive and let it go. Tapping into new memories of my mom and giving her permission to share her spirit allowed me to craft a picture of Mom with wings on my right shoulder to look over me. The energy I feel from her makes me smile and reminds me I'm loved.

Learning more about food, the power and meaning of ingredients, and how they create different reactions was important. The certified intuitive food therapist teachings trained me to tap into the instinctive aspect of foods. I used to eat for the wrong reasons, and training changed my mindset. Pulling cards helps me understand what's happening emotionally and intuitively and the foods I should eat to give me the energy and vibe needed to support the actions. Today, I use many healing foods on my health journey: herbs, teas, and phytonutrient lozenges for healing options (when needed), journaling, and oracle cards for clarity.

Cravings have been one of my teachers all along.

THE TOOL

Before you start this section, grab a piece of paper, find a quiet place, light a candle, and play some soft music. Permit yourself to express your thoughts and feelings on paper. Take some time for this exercise; don't rush.

What do you think, feel, see, taste, or smell when you think about the word craving? Your mental state affects everything around food and your cravings, promoting health or emotional sickness. How would you describe your mental state at this time? Have you thought about what your body says about the foods you crave? What else you might be dealing with that could cause good or bad choices? What does your body need? It could be the same thing, but our cravings often try to tell us something if we pay attention. Cravings come from what is happening in your life, feelings, and emotions. They can trigger different questions both emotionally and physically. They might have different needs in your body.

I will focus on three different cravings that people experience. Foods associated with that craving, diagnoses a doctor would give related to the craving, and alternative solutions to swap the craving for something healthy.

Sugar is the number one craving.

Foods you may think of:

Cookies, ice cream, candy, desserts, etc.

Health issues the doctor might have talked with you about:

Joint pain, swelling, bloating, weight gain, acne, mood swings, irritability, lack of energy, tossing and turning at night, craving more sugar, having a headache, and snapping at people.

What could be some solutions on your own?

Ask yourself if you've eaten a well-balanced meal recently.

Your body might be out of fuel. Choose good fats high in omega-3 fatty acids and protein like salmon, olive oil, and avocados.

What's happening emotionally?

Do you need a sugar or dopamine hit when your world turns upside down? Choose a song, soft music, a quiet place, smell a scent, get some fresh air, or maybe a nap.

When this is the case, you don't usually need food. Try drinking water to hydrate or get some sleep. It usually does the trick!

Don't think about it—keep writing. This helps your brain process what happens in your subconscious.

At first, it'll be slow, but don't be afraid to start. You'll write poems and songs and allow your creativity to flow.

Allow your mind and soul to accept what comes.

You're doing this for yourself to be healthier and work through pain and guilt (or whatever else is ready to release). Let it out.

This is what is making you sick, and you want to let it go and be healthy.

Pay attention to the foods that are lower in calories. Sometimes, they add sugar and aren't always healthier.

Start to swap out foods.

Starting with some simple changes, you must figure out what you want to start with until you can make it a habit. Apples are easy to take with you in your bag and have on hand. Some are soft or crispy, sweet or tart. Find the one you like.

Add some peanut butter without sugar to get some fats and protein.

Dates and pecans together taste like pecan pie. Dates with pecan or peanuts and chocolate drizzled with chocolate on the top taste like a healthy snicker bar.

Roasted sweet potatoes and pumpkin with cinnamon and a teaspoon of maple syrup are also a delicious choice.

Salty is your craving?

Foods you would think of:

Potato chips, pretzels, and corn chips.

Health issues the doctor might have talked with you about:

You have increased thirst, swollen feet or hands, headache (in some cases), and a rise in blood pressure.

Salt induces your hypothalamus to release dopamine.

The signs of dehydration: are dry mouth, feeling weak, fatigue, irritability, and headache.

What could be some solutions on your own?

Depending on your activity level, you might need some electrolytes. To make some drinks on your own, you can add pink or Celtic salt to your water with lemon or lime to make your sports drink.

You might just need sleep.

Some salty processed foods also have sugar in them to trick you. Read the labels.

Healthier swaps:

Consider celery, salty nuts, string cheese, beef jerky, and cheese with mustard because these options provide some fat and salt without the need for chips.

Make crackers with flaxseeds and spices.

Roasted vegetables with olive oil and salt, garlic, paprika, old bay.

Fatty foods:

Foods you would think of:

Fast foods, popcorn, cheese crackers, cakes, pastries, pies, salad dressing, and ice cream.

Health issues the doctor might have talked with you about: Bloating, stomach pain, diarrhea, weight gain, obesity, increased risk of heart disease, stroke, risk of diabetes, acne, and impaired brain function.

Good fats: Olive oil, seeds, fish, avocados, chia seed, flaxseed, hard-boiled eggs, walnuts, pecans, almonds (roast them for a better taste), hummus, tuna.

Make flaxseed crackers.- follow me on Pinterest for recipes-

Use olive oil and a splash of lemon for your salad dressing.

Remember to take baby steps forward and create a habit. Make sure you have some snacks with you at all times so you don't resort to fast food or know what the better options are when you eat out.

Be proud of yourself for taking the time to do this exercise. What did you learn about yourself? Did you see a pattern starting? Do you see things you are doing and want to change? Things don't become a habit until we do them for over three weeks. Journal your experience and what you would like to do differently today and tomorrow that you didn't do yesterday. Take time to journal three things positive from today at the end of the day so you can focus on the positive. Repeat this exercise to help you see your triggers with stress. Things could be from your work, or there could be things from home that you want to change. You'll look back three to six months from today, realizing that what you learned today has been the turning point for making better food and emotional choices.

Swapping foods will take a little planning for meals and healthy snacks. Better nutritional options will help to reduce your cravings for sugar, salt, and fatty foods. Hydration is critical to reduce cravings. Suppose you're drinking twelve ounces of water today; tomorrow, up your game to twenty-four until you get to sixty- four ounces. Start experimenting with cooking, but start with a few easy recipes with readily available ingredients. Crackers are one recipe with flaxseeds, chia seeds, salt, and spice, which is one bowl and spread on a cookie sheet. Permit yourself to succeed, not the option to fail.

Do you need to change the pictures you have in your memories? Do you need to love your inner child from a painful memory you had? I'd love for you to reach out to me if something in my story touched your life and if you need a turnaround experience from sad to happy. I want to celebrate with you! I'd love to be your cheerleader for the smallest change you make. You need someone in your corner, and I'd love to be that person.

Loving my past and knowing what I worked through to heal myself emotionally, physically, spiritually, and mentally helped me help others love their inner child and realize food is healing—things we crave can be life-changing.

I wish you the best on your journey.

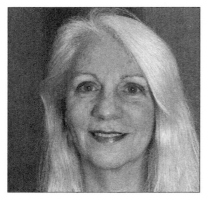

Linda McBee. Helping people with their health and navigating life has become Linda's passion since being a teen, both personally and professionally, working with businesses alongside having her own. Cooking exceptional food became her expression. Keeping it simple with spices is her passion. Growing up in a garden, eating fresh vegetables, and learning to compost to restore the nutrients in the soil is critical. Linda believes giving soil extra nutrients is like taking herbs and botanicals to boost the food we eat. She teaches through experience and explains how trying to eliminate gluten and other chemicals was a good start, and sourcing herbs and additional nutrients to help her cells heal has been a journey. Autoimmune issues are something she's been battling since she was young. Over time snowballed into being diagnosed with neurological Lyme disease. Finding herbs and phytonutrients, her body didn't reject was critical in the search for better health. Linda was fortunate to be introduced to a full line of botanicals a few years ago that are lozenges and have been game-changers. One of them addresses gut issues and eliminating parasites, which was a lifesaver for her journey, ridding her of the brain fog, being sick every time she ate, and increasing her energy level to get back to life again. Another for pre-work and stamina. The latest addresses visceral fat, which is a silent killer, and high in B vitamins. This has been critical since she doesn't assimilate Vitamin B and now can because of the delivery system.

Linda works with individuals, coaches, weight loss centers, wellness centers, practitioners, and mental health centers, directing them around health and loving their inner child to be their best version of themselves.

She'd love to cheer you on your health journey. Please reach out to her at:

https://linktr.ee/LindaMcBee

CHAPTER 8

YOGIC REMEDY FOR THE PERFECTIONIST

A PROFOUND FORGIVENESS PATH FOR SELF-WORTH RETRIEVAL

Julianne Bushnell-Farrell

MY STORY

My heart races and I white knuckle grip the steering wheel. My brain goes on autopilot, and I slam the brakes to a halt in the middle of an intersection in rush hour traffic! Heaviness from the tail end of my soccer mom's minivan launches me forward from the sheer velocity of the stop! I hear myself shriek, "They're getting away!" like a good cop defeated from a high-speed chase. I'm wide awake as if plucked from a dream. *What? Huh? Me?* I'm panting frantically.

A sobering inner voice rams my senses much the same as a critical finger jammed into my chest: *Yes, you!*

Fully present, I skillfully reverse the van towards the crosswalk like a little girl reaching into the forbidden cookie jar before dinner.

My eyes dart left, then right. *Have I been seen?* I silently reassure my shaken inner child. *No one must know!* The van creeps back to an acceptable distance at the crosswalk like a lid returning atop the cookie jar.

No one must know of this or my other road rage experiences! This one occurred after I dropped the kids off at school on carpool day. The behavior eventually bubbled everywhere—anger with my husband, children, parents, friends, and career. *No, not the career!* The one thing in my life I was excellent at was planning multitudes of high-end events and weddings. The place where I'm ultimately in control of every last detail and fulfill my inner perfectionist! I made dreams come true and connected to the most important moments of people's lives. I prided myself on being the best, rarely making mistakes for years! I was disciplined, hard-working, and self-sacrificing for the utmost perfection. Event and wedding planning in Chicago for over twenty years made me a hard egg to crack. However, do you know the old English nursery rhyme of Humpty Dumpty? He sat on a wall and had a big fall! My wall of control soon came crumbling down.

The present moment is the perfect teacher.

~ Baron Baptiste

One evening after a long week, I was doing housework while multitasking children's activities, meals, bath time, etc., in perfect, perfectionist fashion. Suddenly, I had another wake-up call. I remember asking my little one to do a chore. Eagerly, they ran off to do so. An hour went by. I was up to my ears still multitasking, neglecting my needs in the basic ways (diet, exercise, sleep, and even holding off on using the restroom) so I could cross more things off the list!

While stocking the fridge, I felt tired, hungry, resentful, and was still trying to get organized before I could settle down. I heard a voice inside egging me on: *You know you are the only one that can do this right!* Suddenly, my little one slid across the kitchen floor for a snack.

Annoyed, I asked, "Honey, have you completed the chore I gave you yet?"

"Yes, Mommy!"

Unsatisfied, the authoritarian within me prods, "Honey, are you sure it's done perfectly?" I repeat, "Perfffffecttttt?"

Silence.

Time stands still. The hairs on the back of my neck stand on end.

Squatting at the fridge door, I turn eye to eye with my beloved child, thinking: *What did I just say? How could I?* Their soul looked right through mine as if asking the same questions.

I salvage any last bit of grace and softly say, "I mean, the best you can do, Honey!"

I placed this crucial parenting mistake into the growing bag of emotional bypassing I carried since childhood.

From an early teen, I remember my peer group feeding this false imagery of perfectionism.

A shrill school bell rings. The screech of desk chairs scrape the floor. The entire class launches for the exit door into the hallway. Dakota Junior High hallways were where all the action lived in between classes. Older grades dominated the top floor—it was the best! You could see the latest fads and teen romances, hear music, and buy candies, gum, speed, weed, and other recreational drugs. Absent-mindedly, I rushed down the hallway, crashing into a popular school jock of the ninth grade. He looked me up and down, then directly in my eyes, and defiantly asked, "Who are you?"

Barely audible and shaking in my seventh-grade shoes, I reply, "Julie." I'm too shy in my youth to use the full name of Julianne.

"Julie, what?" the arrogant teen asks.

"Julie Bushnell!" I self-consciously chirp. He laughed out loud with a look of shock, "What? Are you telling me you are related to Lisa Bushnell?"

I shook my head yes and pridefully said, "That's my sister."

He called over his buddies and asked if they believed what I said. They also looked me up and down mockingly and laughed! With disbelief, the lead jock inquired, "Are you sure?"

Before I could answer, he hit his closest buddy in the chest and laughed, "You look nothing like her!"

Most people in our rural community knew of my older sister—her reputation as a small-town model and badass beauty prevailed wherever I went. A taunting laughter burst out in the gathering crowd at the scene. He yelled in my face, "Bullshit!" and coolly strode away.

The laughing crowd seemed to close in. Red-faced and disheartened, I raced out of the area. I felt the sting of shame and embarrassment. This wasn't my first demeaning incident, yet the hardest to swallow for being compared to a "perfect model of beauty," my sister (by our community standards). I swallowed my tears and buried this worthiness wound deep within. I told no one. I measured and compared myself from that day forward to others on a rating of beauty, body image, popularity, intelligence, materialism, grit, badassery, etc.

Am I enough? This question deeply embedded its fangs into my framework and repeated through my inner dialogue for years. By age 40, my body hurt, and my moon cycle was erratic. Mentally, I experienced memory lapses where I couldn't remember what I was saying in mid-sentence. My brain was overloaded from multitasking, trying to be the badass, a superwoman who could do everything. Outbursts were more common. I was never to blame! Everyone else was!

I close the door behind me to sit on the patio swing alone. Once again, resisting any sense of responsibility for my perfectionist, snarky actions has created cyclical work drama. My husband is tired of hearing me rationalize my guilt. So there I sulk, alone on the patio swing. *You are the problem!* I hear the dark shadow from within. *You have always been the problem!* Nauseating sensations of shame flood my solar plexus. *Everyone knows you are the problem - work, family, friends, and now you sit alone! You are not worthy to have their love!*

A harsh gust from the north grabs my attention. The cold north wind plummets directly into my chest. I lose my breath. Within a moment, the south wind joins its counterpart. I fall back into the north wind's grip. I'm tossed from left to right and receive blows from each side like a boxing match. A howl as loud as a freight train squalls with tornado-like force. All directions: east, west, north, and south winds whip through the yard. Paper, leaves, refuse scurry to hide from the wind's wrath. I shield my eyes from flying debris and bury my face in my knees. Thoughts teem down like pouring rain.

Am I seeing this for real? A furious blast out of nowhere! It's happening so fast. Why now?

A magnificent rainbow of sheer knowing washes over my entire being like calm after a storm. At that moment, I know with complete clarity that the helix of wind is the Holy Spirit! A message from the Divine! My spine goes erect. I embrace the force of the fierce winds without fear. I taste the salty tears of acceptance rolling down my face.

Yes, I receive you, Holy Spirit! I am open to your guidance. I want to heal myself! I want my family to heal!

The wind storm retracted as fast as it came. I'm in awe and left in stillness from my resonating truth. *I'm willing to change!*

> *I don't think there is anything braver than forgiveness.*
>
> ~ Brene Brown

Enter yoga. From the first class, I was hooked! I discovered the meaning of letting go, from the simplicity of breath to the depths of my spirit—a hole in one!

The warm, golden flicker of candlelight greets me as I enter the hot yoga room. Over the next hour, I journey into listening, finally releasing control. I can get into many postures. I even dare to view my body in the mirror and peer into my eyes. I simmer into a hip opener on the right side near the end of class. I settle onto my forearms and melt down into the stillness. I hear the instructor's gentle voice say one word: "Forgiveness." Internally, I feel a tingling in my ears from the vibrational tone of the word.

The instructor delicately continues with self-inquiry, "How does forgiveness play out in your life?" leaving space for the past to come forth. My mind toggles with the career, the superficial layers, the conflicts, and the triggers. I question if I can forgive the toxicity of my current working conditions. I still myself and listen to the possibility of absolution present.

Another soft prompt, "Whom do you need to forgive?" Layers open to my husband, siblings, and parents. I reflect. With my head down, sweat dripping, I forgive each person for past experiences I deemed wrong. I feel an energetic release in the heart with each pardon.

I listen as the teacher of life returns her disciple's attention to their anatomy for the left side of the pose. Silently, I dissolve into the parameters of my body and crave more spiritual inquiry. In a few minutes, I hear a whisper in my left ear, "I encourage you to let go now, deeper into your exhalations, and forgive yourself." My body liquefies on the mat. *Could my spirit be directly spoken to in a yoga class?* It had been so long since I experienced the soulful truth reverberating through my cells. An electric pulse floods warmth and light sensations through my heart, the return of Self. *The first stages of self-worth retrieval!*

In that *aha* moment, I forgive myself for not living up to the demands of perfectionism. I feel deep disappointment for not meeting the expectations of my loved ones and colleagues. Salty tears flow. The burden of carrying this emotional weight is released. *Yes, I can forgive myself for making past mistakes!*

Pure magic, all from the sacredness of a yoga mat! A down-up approach—body, mind, spirit. My yoga practice expanded to a safe space to release pent-up energy, emotions, body tension, and mental stress while receiving higher consciousness. The yogic philosophy of "the God within" blows my mind every time I step on a mat to give or receive—reciprocity. People come to the mat for inspiration or desperation. I received both. The mat became my mirror. A reflection of my external world from observing my inner dialogue on the mat.

Yoga is defined as yoke or union. This yoke can be practicing postures on a mat, in one's breath, through stillness, reading, pen to paper, walking, playing or listening to music, and countless other forms of body, mind, and spirit union.

I had no idea yoga would be the catalyst to living my dreams. I've learned to embrace my fear, challenge my perspective, and parent my inner child while sharing my heart with humans, plants, and animals—the most important job I've had. What an honor to guide others through the medicine of oneness. The medicinal soul journey of self-love. *The ability to know thyself, love thyself, through thyself.*

Over the years, this awakening didn't come easy. I felt confused between the two voices in my head from adolescence through adulthood. The soft, gentle deer voice is always more receptive, and the fierce lioness voice fights for my personal power. It was a battle over whom to listen to and whom to trust. One is anger, resentment, jealousy, self-pity, guilt, inferiority, superiority, and ego. The other is peace, love, humility, kindness, empathy, patience, compassion, and surrender. The inner conflict on which was right or wrong laid the perfect groundwork for a consistent yoga practice. When the mind serves the body, the soul emerges.

"If we want to love, we must learn how to forgive."

~ Mother Teresa

Your body is a house, a temple of divinity. It knows exactly what to do and when to do it! It's filled with infinite, cosmic intelligence far beyond our present state of consciousness.

The body never lies. The secret is to listen! Pay attention to the signs, signals, and subtle clues it gives of universal truth. The truth will reveal what voice within you to feed: the voice of love (the gentle deer) or the voice of fear (the fierce lion).

When grounded into our physical body, the mind serves the body, and the Self rises. In this seat of the highest Self, wisdom is clear. The wisdom or intuition feels calm and balanced. Connection to the whole (oneness) versus separation. Feelings are the energetic sensations that flow through your body. The communication from your body. It's hard to hear what your body says when your mind has 60,000+ thoughts daily. It's easy to become distracted by these thoughts and disconnect from the signals of universal intelligence within our physical body. The lion becomes present for purpose, navigation, and reflection of what exists underneath the surface level. The true emotion we're protecting ourselves from. Emotion means energy in motion. Emotional feelings are meant to be felt and then released. No harm, no judgment, no attachment. The opposite of carrying decades of emotional baggage and embodied unworthiness.

The gateway to return to the body and the wisdom of our highest Self is through two simple yet life-giving actions: movement synced with breath in the present moment!

THE TOOL

PROGRESSIVE WORTHINESS MEDITATION

Breath - your inhalation is the inspiration. Your exhalation is letting go, to forgive.

1. Sit or lay in a comfortable position.

2. Place one hand on your belly and one hand on your heart.

3. Breathe from your belly up to your heart space.

4. Breathe out from your heart space down to your belly.

5. Inhale - inflate your belly up to your heart.

6. Exhale - deflate from your heart to your belly.

7. Lower your hands to your lap. Breathe in. Shrug your shoulders to your ears. Squeeze up. Hold your breath in for a slow ten-count.

8. Breathe out. Drop your shoulders. Let go of the pent-up energy. Close your eyes. Observe the flood of release through your upper body. Breathe naturally and sit for a few moments.

9. Inhale deeply, hold your breath, and make fists with your hands and feet. Hug your finger/toe knuckles close to your palms/ball mount of your feet, respectively. Grip tight and hold for a slow count of ten.

10. Now exhale and release your finger and toe grips completely. Close your eyes and relinquish control for a minute or two.

11. Squish your face up as if eating a sour lemon. Close your eyes, wrinkle your forehead and nose. Pucker your lips like no one is watching. Take a big breath and hold. Pucker more for a slow ten count.

12. Exhale. Relax your face. Enjoy the natural sensations of releasing tension through your facial muscles. Soak in the liberation.

13. Wrap your non-dominant arm under the dominant one for a bear hug. Pull your hip bones in towards each other. Engage your buttocks to your sit bones. Fill your lungs with air as best you can and compress inward. Hold for a slow ten-count. Take another sip in. Hold for two more counts.

14. Exhale deeply, releasing all the activation in your body. Breathe naturally and sit in your vitality. Embrace the free-flowing energy coursing through your body.

15. Pucker your face, bear hug with the dominant arm under, shrug your shoulders to your ears, and squeeze your toes, buttocks, and hips together at the same time. Inhale a gigantic breath. Hold for a slow ten-count. Sip in more air. Hold for five more counts! Yes, you can!

16. Breathe out, let go, and soften every part of your body. Sit for as long as you like, liberated from the seat of Source, and absorb your worthiness!

17. Layer your hands on your belly. Inhale and declare with each exhaling breath "I am worthy"! Proclaim three times with breath. Open your eyes and proceed on a life centered in self-worth!

HO'OPONOPONO PRAYER ~ AN ANCIENT HAWAIIAN PRACTICE OF FORGIVENESS

I'm Sorry

Please forgive me

Thank you

I love you

The prayer intends to reconcile, restoring balance and self-love.

The word ho'oponopono means to remedy what is wrong or cause a return to balance. The prayer is chanted repeatedly to cleanse the body of ill will and negative feelings.

Profound self-forgiveness comes when you stand in the emotional trigger and parent the inner child from the worthiness of your soul.

1. Practice the meditation above. Close your eyes. Place your hands on your heart.

2. Visualize yourself as a child (clothing, hair, facial expression in an activity you loved to do).

3. Look directly into the eyes of your inner child. Kindly say, *"I Love You."*

4. Receive this love in the depths of your heart.

5. Sincerely say, "I'm Sorry." Acknowledge the hurt you have endured, a specific wound or collective wounds.

6. Accept your apology.

7. Considerately say, "Please forgive me" for not awakening earlier to the pattern or experience.

8. Embrace the realization of breaking free from a karmic cycle.

9. Thoughtfully say, " Thank You" for enduring the journey you have lived through.

10. Repeat these four mantras 108 times. Add mala beads for accountability of the 108 repetitions.

11. This prayer also can be utilized to forgive others.

**Hear audible versions of the forgiveness practices at
www.thehouseofwellnessbyjulianne.com/youareworthit.**

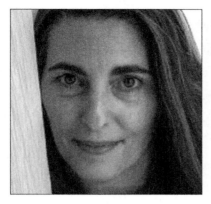

Julianne Farrell, E-RYT 500 | AYS | RMS | CYPT | CYLC | YACEP found her way from the sacred Black Hills of South Dakota to the fast pace of Chicago's event industry after graduating college with a business degree in hospitality. She spent 25 years catering to others in luxury accommodations with hours on her feet and too much time behind a computer. The stress experienced led her to passionately pursue personal wellness as a call to action! This action led her to share her knowledge and intuitive techniques in all aspects of wellness for everyone!

Julianne is a certified E-RYT 500-Hour Yoga/meditation instructor, Reiki Master, sound therapist, Ayurveda Yoga Specialist, and Yoga Alliance Continuing Education Provider.

She is deeply honored to guide others into the resonance of Yoga, balance, energy, and sound healing to relieve stress, anxiety and pain, while supporting expansion.

She's the founder of The House of Wellness, a nurturing space dedicated to private healing through yoga, Reiki, and sound therapy. She's taught, mentored, and administered healing practices in Chicagoland and the nation. She's planned and executed events from the hospitality industry to the wellness world. On international platforms (live & virtual), national retreats, training/wellness programs, and intimate healing circles. Her passion is connection, fostering community, and harmonizing group consciousness. When we heal, the earth heals.

Her work is featured on two personal wellness app virtual platforms: Chill Anywhere and The Rate App.

Julianne loves a good cup of tea, cats, and travel! Whether a beachside Yoga studio, mom-and-pop diner, or an adventure into the beauty of Mother Gaia, you can find Julianne celebrating the present moment!

Connect with Julianne Farrell for Therapeutic Services:

Website: https://www.thehouseofwellnessbyjulianne.com

Facebook: https://www.facebook.com/julianne.farrell.5

Instagram: https://www.instagram.com/thehouseofwellnessbyjulianne/

Email: thehouseofwellnessbyjulianne@gmail.com

CHAPTER 9

RAISE THE VIBRATION OF THE FOOD YOU EAT

TRANSMUTING TOXINS AND POLLUTANTS WITH THE VIOLET FLAME

Angela Orora Medway-Smith, The Practical Mystic

"Let food be thy medicine
And medicine be thy food."

~ Hippocrates

MY STORY

My usual psychic protection failed, and I felt, heard, and re-lived the experience of the animals whose remains graced the pristine white shelves, packed into small trays covered in clingfilm.

I stood statue still.

Beads of cold sweat rolled down my forehead as my entire body froze in fear.

Nausea rose in my gut.

I heard screams and felt as if I'd been shoved into a tiny space; the noise was deafening.

"Are you okay?" a voice echoed, sounding far away; I felt a touch on my arm.

I broke from what felt like a trance of terror and turned my head.

"Yes, thank you. I just felt unwell for a moment. I'll be fine," I replied to the concerned passer-by.

I was in the supermarket picking up something for dinner and wandered into the meat aisle.

I stepped away, looking for a chair so I could compose myself.

Dear Lord! This has never happened before, so why now?

My guides responded clearly.

Your vibration is high, and you can no longer consume animal flesh.

For months, I strayed away from meat, only consuming tiny amounts when cooking meals for my family, choosing plant protein sources instead, an anathema to my carnivore husband.

Even when absentmindedly snacking during meal preparation, my gut responded with nausea when meat got close to my lips; I was reminded that my body rejected it.

This was the final message. *No meat.*

I already had some dietary challenges, juvenile diabetes, celiac disease, and a host of allergies.

In the 21st century, surely eliminating meat couldn't be that difficult.

It became apparent that, in most restaurants in my town, you could be vegetarian or vegan, but not celiac and vegetarian, and have a choice of meals.

My food choices when eating out were mushroom risotto or chickpea curry. Cooking for my family wasn't a problem; everything was celiac-friendly anyway. I just changed my protein source.

Or so I thought.

As the months rolled by, I noticed my clothes getting tighter as the pounds piled on.

My physical fitness deteriorated as I made fatty dairy choices (cheese is my nemesis) and added quick, pre-packaged vegetarian products to the healthy, balanced meals I cooked for my family.

My work as an energy healer, spiritual teacher, and channel for the Ascended Master and Archangelic collectives moved on at a pace. I channeled books, an Atlantean healing modality, and guidance for thousands of people, my connections crystal clear as I consumed only high-vibrational foods.

However, I was finding it increasingly difficult to maintain a healthy weight without access to low-fat animal proteins, and by this point, I had put on almost 60 pounds.

So, sitting in meditation, I asked my guides:

Will eating fish affect my vibration?

No, providing you transmute any negative vibrations and toxins with the violet flame, it will be well.

Slowly and carefully, I reintroduced small amounts of fish into my diet. I already blessed my food and gave gratitude to every being that brought my meal to me; I simply needed to add another small step and transmute all that didn't serve me from the contents of the plate.

Within weeks, I noticed a difference. My skin, hair, and nails had more clarity, shine, and strength, but the pounds remained. I accepted that perhaps, in my fifties, this was now my shape. I was far too busy to pay any more attention to my body.

Seven years passed after my experience in the supermarket, and I received instruction from my guides:

You will travel to the Temple of Hathor and reopen the energetic portal to the Pleiades.

I was shown my past life, in which I served at this temple, assisting people in physically traveling through this portal.

I don't argue with my guides anymore when given such instructions. They always create a clear path to enable me to carry out the work they ask for.

I opened my phone, and almost immediately, a post popped up. A friend in Glastonbury was leading a pilgrimage to the temples of the Nile. I messaged her, arranging to meet for coffee a few days later.

"You have the last place, Angela," she smiled.

"We knew something special would be happening at Hathor's Temple at Dendera, so we booked a private session there after all the tourists leave."

I was absolutely thrilled and looked forward to this once-in-a-lifetime experience.

Aircraft meals are an issue.

You can order vegan, vegetarian, halal, kosher, and celiac food, but not celiac and vegetarian food. On this trip, my travel agent suggested I request halal food as this is often a rice dish.

Unlucky again, I thought as I sent the gluten-containing meal back. The gluten-free option was meat, as usual, and the vegetarian meal was pasta. I dug into my bag for the falafel and gluten-free protein bars I carry as emergency food.

Cairo was insane.

I have no other words to describe it.

It's a dirty, crowded, noisy, smelly, melting pot of humanity; people either love it or hate it.

I hated it.

It overwhelmed my senses.

I was glad to be part of a group on this occasion. It felt as if we were divinely protected.

Our trip to Giza's Great Pyramid during a full moon and solar eclipse was a powerful, unique, and expansive experience.

Our temple pilgrimage was simply incredible. I joined a group of French and Belgian Magdalene priestesses and Templar knights as we re-remembered past lives, received codes of light, and intuitively created energy vortexes and portals as we traveled from Cairo to Aswan together.

After a stay in Luxor, we traveled on a private dahabiya boat and were treated like royalty.

A few days into the trip, we had the opportunity to visit the village of one of the sailors in the Nubian marshes, which is not somewhere tourists usually venture.

The plan was to set out after afternoon tea. Teas and beautiful cakes were laid out. I asked Saïd, our waiter, for my usual banana.

"Sorry, madam, bananas are no good." I nodded sadly.

Oh no! I really needed a banana to fill me up!

The walk in this heat will send me hypo. I'll need to turn off my insulin pump, get an energy bar from my emergency stash, and make sure I've got plenty of dextrose on me.

We set off shortly afterward, a forty-minute dusty walk across the marshes to a small village.

We were warmly welcomed into the sailor's home. We sat in the spartan room on hard wooden pallets, being greeted by a procession of villagers. During the next half an hour, we were given babies to hold, photographed with different groups of locals, and sipped mint tea.

It was a truly humbling experience. Beautiful souls who had so little, offering their friendship and love.

Small boys ran alongside us with flashlights, smiling and chattering, lighting our return to the boat.

Showered and now very hungry, I headed toward the long wooden table on the deck for dinner. It was late, and the delicious smell of fresh-baked bread filled my nostrils as I headed to help myself to soup.

As I lifted the lid of the soup pot, nausea rose in my belly. I smelled chicken.

"Saïd, is there meat in the soup, my friend?" I asked in a panic, stomach growling.

"Yes, madam, it is very fresh, very good."

Crestfallen, I replied sadly, "Many of us do not eat meat."

I took my place at the table, every other person hungrily tucking into the bread and soup as I waited for everyone to finish and the main course to arrive.

Tears welled up in my eyes. I was tired and hungry. Thankfully, my blood glucose levels were okay.

"Why aren't you eating?" a friend asked.

"There's meat in the soup" I replied, and excused myself to hide the tears now beginning to roll down my face.

I moved to the edge of the boat and gazed over the waves gently lapping on the opposite bank of the Nile, the moon shining brightly in the star-filled sky beaming down from above.

This is ridiculous. I'm a grown woman I shouldn't be crying. Get a grip, Angela. There'll be food in about fifteen minutes! I sighed deeply, wiping the salty tears that streamed down my face.

As our main course was laid out, I dashed to fill my plate with rice, vegetables, and my favorite, aubergine.

The following morning, we had time to meditate and journal as the boat sailed gently south. My guides spoke:

You can eat meat now.

What?! How can I eat meat? Even last night, I felt the vibration of the animal in the food.

You can eat meat now. It is done.

How can I be a clear channel if I eat meat again? How will I serve? How can I do my work? I questioned in panic.

You can eat meat now. It is done. If you do not believe us, speak to Eléonore.

My gaze settled on a beautiful French lady at the boat's bow whom I'd spoken to in passing.

Okay, let's hear what she has to say.

Eléonore confirmed something similar happened to her and suggested I take it slowly—not feel any pressure by putting a tiny amount of meat on my plate, and only when I felt able to bring it to my mouth and eat.

My guides clearly altered something energetically in my being to enable me to nourish my body more easily.

I put this to the back of my mind as we made our next stop—to swim in the Nile!

We docked at a small island dotted with local children laughing as they played, splashed, and swam in the clear, fast-flowing water.

Excited, I felt like a child myself; while others stepped tentatively into the cold river, I ran and dived in head first, swimming slightly upriver to float back to the group and repeating this sequence until called for lunch.

I felt incredibly cleansed and energized. It was a magical experience.

It was our last night aboard the boat. Later, at dinner, the head chef appeared for the first time, dressed in pristine whites, a banquet beautifully laid out before us.

This food has been cooked with so much love and pride; this is the best opportunity I'll have to try meat.

I thanked him for all of our wonderful meals, took a deep breath, and nervously put a tiny amount of duck on my plate.

No nausea, that's a good sign.

I sat down at the table next to Eléonore for support. I blessed my food and transmuted any toxins and pollutants with the violet flame.

I was very anxious; I tucked into the vegetables and played with the meat.

Angela, dive in like you did into the Nile today, Cariad, and don't forget to chew 28 times like I taught you! I hear the unmistakable booming voice of my grandfather in my inner ear.

My grandfather passed away when I was fifteen years old, but I'm incredibly blessed that he shows up when I need a nudge.

Okay, Grampie, here goes! I smiled.

I put a tiny shred of meat on my fork and brought it slowly to my mouth.

Nothing except the taste of the meat. No nausea, no horrifying images or feelings. As my guides said, I could eat meat again.

I expected the earth to move at this point, but there was nothing but the sound of the water, the chatter of my fellow diners, and Grampie's smiling face as he left.

Isn't it strange that enormous occurrences for us go unnoticed by others?

They become frozen moments in time.

I'm forever grateful to my guides.

Since that moment, I've listened to my body, choosing only food that nurtures it.

I've changed the vibration of the foods I eat to ensure that my energetic body, spirit, and physical body are nurtured and nourished.

It's a simple process that I'm blessed to share with you now.

THE TOOL

Everything we put into or on our body holds a vibration that can affect us in both a positive and negative way.

It was Nikola Tesla who said, "If you want to find the secrets of the universe, think in terms of energy, frequency, and vibration."

If you want to cherish your body temple, it makes sense to consume high-vibrational food and drink. This can be challenging for many people, especially if you're away from home.

Most of the time, we have no idea of the energetic food chain that has created the meal that's put in front of us.

Was it created with high vibrational elements? With love and integrity?

So, if we can't ensure that it has, we can use this simple process to change that.

To infuse the love of the divine into the food on our plates and transmute any toxins or pollutants that have entered the food chain.

There are many prayers and sacred symbols that can change the vibration of the food you eat.

I'll be writing about them in detail in my forthcoming book series with Lainie Sevanté Wulkan, the first of which *Angelic Resonance* will be published later in 2024.

Here, I'm sharing a simple prayer and the sacred symbol of the violet flame to specifically transmute the toxins and pollutants that might be present in your food.

I'm a light trance channel for the Ascended Master St. Germain, who guards and guides the violet flame. I teach others how to access and harness its power from all dimensions, bringing the gifts of higher clairvoyance and powerful healing rescue flames.

We have access to many sacred flames and esoteric energies for our spiritual development and healing. You can find more information in my channeled books *The Book of Many Colours: Awaken Your Soul's Purpose With The Divine Rays* and *The Book of Many Flames: Everyday Alchemy With Esoteric Energies*.

The violet flame is a powerful esoteric energy that exists in every sphere and dimension. It can be invoked to purify and eliminate negative energy across various realms:

- In the physical sphere, it transforms toxins and pollutants.
- In the mental and emotional spheres, it transmutes negative thought, forms and emotions.
- In the spiritual sphere, it cleanses dark spiritual energies like demonic infestation and pollution.

Its sacred symbol, which we use to draw in the power of the violet flame, is a violet seven-pointed star.

THE PRAYER AND VISUALIZATION

Beloved, creator of all that there is,

Thank you for providing me with this nourishment.

I'm grateful for this food and all the beings whose energy and essence brought this meal to my table.

May it strengthen my body and energize my heart, mind, and spirit.

May any energy on this plate that does not serve my highest good be transmuted and every molecule be filled with your divine light.

Next, visualize a violet seven-pointed star* over your plate and push the star image downwards so that any toxins or pollutants in your food are transmuted by the power of the violet flame.

Beloved, bless this meal, in your name which is love,

Amen

*A beautiful image of the violet seven-pointed star that can be printed off and laminated (if you'd like to use it as a table mat) can be downloaded from my website, together with a daily invocation calling in the power of the violet flame for holistic well-being. Find them here:

https://www.cariadspiritual.com/high-vibrational-eating-gift

If you wish to use your own prayer, you can; our words contain powerful intent; simply begin by using my prayer as a guide.

The violet flame is an enormously powerful transformational and transmutational frequency that can change your life in ways you'd never imagined.

I hope my simple little tool brings you abundant health, and high-vibrational wellness.

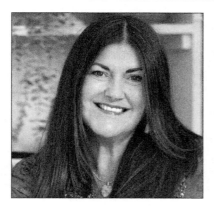

Angela Orora Medway-Smith, "The Practical Mystic," is a Welsh spiritual channel and teacher, master healer, coach, and retreat leader. Her business is called Cariad Spiritual, and she works both in person and online, spreading the light at workshops, festivals, and retreats worldwide.

Holistic healing is Angela's passion. She's Chair of a non-profit, Divine Energy International, dedicated to promoting energy healing and supporting healers of various modalities.

She's set up healing clinics, created charity holistic events and festivals, trained hundreds of energy healers, and supported thousands of clients worldwide with healing and guidance from spirit.

She devotes her life to awakening divine souls like you to their potential. She believes that we all can transform, emerge from the chrysalis of this human life, 'be the butterfly,' and soar, reclaiming our sovereign self, developing a deep connection to our soul, and aligning with our true destiny.

Angela is incredibly blessed to be a direct channel for the angelic realm and Ascended Masters. She has published two channeled books *The Book of Many Colours: Awaken Your Soul's Purpose With The Divine Rays* and *The Book of Many Flames: Everyday Alchemy With Esoteric Energy.*

She's also co-author of five number-one international Amazon best-selling books on holistic healing, all of which you can find here: https://www.amazon.co.uk/stores/Angela-Orora-Medway-Smith/author/B09L5X6T7X

Angela offers spiritual consultations, coaching, mentoring, retreats, healing, healer, and intuitive development training worldwide.

She loves to empower others to kick-start their healing journey and spiritual development.

When she's not supporting others or with her family, you'll find Angela by water, walking along the banks of the Thames, which flows near her London home, or along the beach close to her hometown in Wales.

Connect with Angela at:

https://linktr.ee/angela_orora_medwaysmith

Remember to sign up for her newsletter to receive monthly gifts and news.

CHAPTER 10

DIVINE FEMININE EMERGENCE

HEART CONSCIOUS CONNECTION
TO HONORING YOUR TRUTH

Susan G. Chamberlain, Ph.D.,
Ancient Mystic Soul Transformation

*"Remember that nothing is small in the eyes of GOD.
Do all that you do with love."*

~ Saint Therese of Lisieux

MY STORY

So there it was, staring me in the face, bold and loud. Right in the middle of Central Park, in the blazing sunlight, I had a huge aha moment, an epiphany. A whole new reality set in. I had to leave my career of 34 years. I called my sister Cindy immediately. "Your path is being redirected on purpose by the hand of GOD, she exclaimed." I felt hot and cold at the same time. Her words protruded through the phone and hit my soul like thorns in my side. I had no groundbreaking plan running through the scope of my mind. Thoughts were running rampant as if someone was chasing them with fire. A rapid pulse coursed through my veins as my eyes got wider.

I dedicated the last 34 years of my life to helping others. As a medical professional in a 555-bed hospital, I felt all alone after being surrounded by so many others. The patients became my lifeline in so many fulfilling ways. This career filled my heart and soul with joy, as I always felt like Mother Teresa. She followed her soul path, and now I am going to follow mine.

I felt a deeper calling. It was time for me to move on to my spiritual work, the work I knew only my soul could do. This sometimes left me paralyzed with fear as to how I'd begin. And now it's happening.

My ego wants to feel safe. It likes to keep me small, unseen, unheard, and unknown. I drifted back in my mind's eye to where my wake-up call pulled me from my daily life. In the mid-1990s, I had H. Pylori. Helicobacter pylori is a bacteria that causes stomach ulcers. This illness was relentless. I wasn't a very good patient since I was never really sick. The formula to get better (four strong medications with milk four times daily for two weeks) nearly wiped me out. Eventually, I completed the two-week regime, but then my normal flora (the body's immune lining) flipped inside out, leaving me with massive sensitivities. I lost my hearing for a year. Cataracts appeared in my eyes for three years. I couldn't walk a straight line. Anything I put into my hands dropped to the ground. My diet changed in one day, from eating everything to eating nothing.

My nourishment is set by divine design by my intuitive vibration, confirmed by Edgar Cayce, the father of holistic medicine. Through healing my gut, my relationship with God grew immensely. I realized I exhausted the use of physical medicine. I needed an alternative method. I put myself through holistic schooling, earning a PhD in holistic theology. The courses telescoped me into the narrow path of the soul. My ancient mystic came to life again. The healing path of my soul illuminated my courageous journey.

From my studies, both scientifically and spiritually, I knew I was out of balance. I began to become very familiar with spiritual terminology. I discovered we have four bodies (physical, emotional, mental, and spiritual), not one. I now had to deal with balancing each one of these on a personal level. This journey generated roads I would've never traveled.

I experienced more spiritual sightseeing than any time I've spent physically on this planet. My spiritual healing turned on multiple profound sensory perceptions. I often found myself in other dimensions. My reality shifted from physical to spiritual, and I enjoyed it. Profound soul modifications were enlightening my spiritual knowledge. Many times, I was left in awe by spirit. Angels and ascended masters were so often in my space, making me feel like this was normal. Archangel Raphael, Archangel Michael, Yeshua (Jesus), and a few others were in my room each day for my studies. They often astral traveled with me. Each night angels took me out of my bed for more spiritual sightseeing.

When I was five years old, I wanted to be a nun. God has always been part of my life, and I'm grateful I remained faithful to my upbringing. I prayed by the side of my bed at the age of two. I knew even then my strength would come from spiritual connections to prayer. It's as if my soul prepared me for what was coming.

After a period of time, things started to connect. The Akashic record (guide history of your soul) pulled up my ancient mystical self, where I mastered the knowledge of spiritual tools. The gathering of ancient wisdom filled my heart and soul. Through soul magnetics, I now drew other souls who squeaked through time unnoticed to assist me with healing.

I was so much better at this point in time. I gained experience and expanded my soul. I earned over 30 spiritual certifications, master level where required, and felt I was ready to help other souls achieve their goals and regain their lives.

This leads me to a client named Elaine. She was feeling distanced from her life and was looking for a change, and I could help her. She was a divorced mom with a couple of kids and spiraled in overwhelm. Her full-time job was demanding both physically and mentally. She wore exhaustion like people wear dungarees.

She met with me one snowy afternoon in November. She looked rugged for a 39-year-old explaining her circumstances. "I just want my sanity back after the divorce," she proclaimed. She last remembered peace before the day she found her husband of 20 years cheating on her.

I welcomed Elaine by sitting her on a high-back lounge chair and pouring her a warm cup of calming chamomile tea with a twist of lemon. She was on the edge, hanging over the side, with only one hand holding on. A meltdown or even a breakdown was bound to be on her next horizon. In the midst of her life challenge, her nephew, who was three or four years old, was in dire need of open heart surgery. "Will you pray for him?" she asked. She handed me a little wooden cross on which his name was etched.

"Of course," I agreed. The angels heard the request before I even knew they did. I noticed an energy shift as I left the room with the cross and entered a sunlit room. I placed the cross in a round-shaped green globe-like plant. In a matter of minutes, the room turned a shade of emerald green like no other. I tried to clear my vision a few times. My attention was now directed to the wooden cross. Fairies were intently and feverishly working on the cross, buzzing around it like they were carving Mount Rushmore. I've not seen fairies do this before. The energy continued in this haze-like moment and pulled me with a heavenly gaze into my kitchen. My jaw dropped, and my divine eyes appeared with a serene embrace marked by the appearance of Archangel Raphael and his team of six-foot angels.

We have received your message. The little boy will make it through and be just fine.

I steadfastly returned to Elaine and was delighted to inform her of the good news; this would be one less burden for her.

She was overjoyed by the angelic message and the messengers who delivered it as I briefly let her in on the divine moment in the kitchen. She then wanted to know what kind of world I lived in. How could I be so calm and have an experience like this? I shared, "I am very spiritual. This is somewhat normal. My faith, trust, and belief are in God and God alone," I explained, "This world is illusionary, and my heart belongs to Heaven."

She listened intently as I shared about the divine feminine emergence in my life. She was all ears, and without blinking, she leaned back in her chair, put her feet up, and said, "I'm ready for the journey."

I enlightened her with some of my mystical experiences. I spoke about the ancient mystic returning through my Akashic records to heal my soul. I shared the integration of my hospital life with Mother Teresa, transforming it into a spiritual life of fulfillment. I explained using a heart-conscious connection honoring my path of truth to stay in integrity, balanced, congruent, grounded, and aligned. "It's a life-long journey that continues into the afterlife," I explained.

Let's help make the divine heart-conscious connection to honoring your truth. The place in your heart that knows best.

THE TOOL

SETTING UP YOUR SACRED SPACE

- Make yourself comfortable in your own sanctuary space, a space you claim as sacred and holy, wherever that may be.
- Sit or stand on a wool cloth. This aids in your grounding connection to Mother Earth and her many layers and dimensions.
- Silence, holy silence works best for me.
- Music of your choice can be a part of this experience; that is a personal preference.
- Gather sacred objects, crystals, oils, books, cards, stones, etc..
- Use holy water, sage, crystals, divine intentions to clear your space and yourself.
- Do not cross your body in any position (arms, legs, hands, etc.).
- Free yourself of restrictions and allow your body to be present in this sacred space with unrestricted flow.
- Candles can be used (fragrant or non-fragrant), as well as dim lighting, natural sun light, or moon light.

SACRED TIME

- Be in your comfortable sacred space.
- Light candles, music on or off.
- Call in your sacred guides, angels, teachers, saints, sages, and ascended masters.
- Begin to close your eyes calmly and feel peaceful.

- Practice the 6-3-6 ancient breathing technique. Inhale to the count of six, hold to the count of three, exhale to the count of six, and hold to the count of three. Do this six times and relax.

- Place your center of intention on your heart energy and your higher heart (soul heart). Build this energy up by continuing to focus there.

- Place your hands over your heart and higher soul heart (space above your physical heart and below your throat).

- Feel you're becoming one with your sacred space.

- Begin to notice you're floating freely in your space.

- Direct your intention to a day dreaming state, a feeling of being free.

SACRED CONNECTION

- With intentional energy and your imagination, focus on your crown chakra, seventh chakra (top of your head), and intentionally open it. You'll feel a connection here to energy from above. Go higher into the celestial realms way up.

- Take your intentional focused energy and pull it down from your crown, down through your higher soul heart, down through your body to the seat of your soul where you sit. Down to your feet and down to the center of Mother Earth feeling her energy, soils, waters, crystals, and heart beating.

- Grounded in Heaven and on Earth, you are now a conduit between Heaven and Earth. Let the energy flow freely through you. You can feel the flow in your sacred silence, with your eyes closed, floating.

- Hands continue on the heart and higher soul heart.

- As you go deeper into a meditative state, you may see, feel, smell, hear, and sense the presence of angels—your angels, sacred guides, ascended masters, and teachers. They're always around you, but now you're focusing on intending to contact them directly.

- Once you feel or sense the sacred connection, you can begin to work with them by permitting them to assist you here and now. You can say this out loud or silently inside: *I am giving you permission to work with me here and now.*

- Your sacred team loves you and loves that you're reaching out for assistance.
- Each member of your sacred team is designed to help you. Have no worries.
- Begin to notice the sacred space around you with your senses and the air around you.
- You can feel a lot of love pouring over, around, through, in you. It can be quite overwhelming. Sometimes I begin to smile, cry, or laugh.

HEART CONSCIOUS CONNECTION TO HONORING YOUR TRUTH

- Now that you're deep into your meditative state, your spiritual senses have begun activating, animating (coming to life) that which your sensory perception is picking up.
- Observe what's happening. Be observant as to what is being picked up by your perception.
- You may see things. You might hear things. Pay attention to anything that captures your attention spiritually.
- Now is the time to put your questions out there. What do I need to know today? What do I need to know at this moment?
- Your intuition is a high-vibrational magnet. It will draw to you what's needed for you to heal.
- Truth—that which is not false about anything. Truth has no contradiction. The actual truism of something, the factual character of being true. What is personally true for you?
- God is truth. I am divine truth, as I know I'm made in the image and likeness of God, a higher power.
- The Ten Commandments are a truth compass for human morality and integrity, not to lie.
- Your spiritual team will give you answers; some may come with divine timing attached. It'll come in God's time when you gain enough knowledge to handle what was given to you.

- Be open to receiving messages and guidance.

- You can be given a healing formula, path, steps, procedures here in this meditative state. Have a pen and paper by your side, and let it happen.

- Make sure you discern who you received your message or answer from. Ask your spiritual team their names. If I feel something false or not right in my field, I ask it to leave.

Take note that your heart is more conscious and intuitive than your mind.

Like your soul, your heart has 100% memory, and you can draw ancient wisdom forward.

God's divine unconditional love is the greatest love of all. Do your best to feel and receive the connection in this lifetime. We are all divine love and light. Love you all.

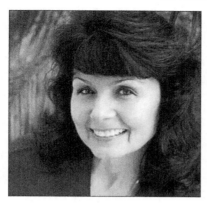

Susan G. Chamberlain, Ph.D. is the founder of Blue Rose Mystics. She is the author of *Holy Quotes from Heaven's Holy Notes, Reclaiming your Soul's Light, Divine Path... Sacred Love...*, 365-day inspirational books, and *33 Seeds of Grace* a prayer book, and International best-selling Co-Author of *Mindset Mastery for Entrepreneurs*. She was also an International Published Article Writer for "Luminous Women' a spiritual magazine.

She was always fascinated by biology while growing up. She holds an A.A.S. degree in clinical medical technology and a B.S. in biology from CUNY City University of New York, The College of Staten Island. Her career was serving others, which she did for 34 years at the same hospital.

She also obtained a degree in holistic theology and went on to her Ph.D. She obtained over 30 spiritual healing certifications, master level on many, while on her path to wellness and wholeness. All were intentional to balance her body, mind, spirit and soul.

She has been professed as a Monk in Celebrating Life Ministries, where she is also an Ordained Minister of Enlightened Spiritual Healing.

She was the host, producer, and director of her own local cable television show in New York *Spirituality Plus* where she interviewed guests.

She now does expo's, workshops, and retreats in NY, NJ, CT, PA, NH, FL. She locally works out of Fairy Dust Crystals & Such offering workshops, lectures, Sarah healing sessions, readings, spiritual Sound Baths.

Susan G. Chamberlain, PhD.

Blue Rose Mystics

https://susangchamberlain.com

https://bit.ly/holynotes

https://linktr.ee/BlueRoseMystics

CHAPTER 11

THE BEING BREATH

CULTIVATING YOUR NATURAL RHYTHM FOR LIFE

Kandy Taylor Love, Child of the Divine

*The Yogis of ancient times wondered: If the condition of the
mind is affecting one's breath, is it possible to change
the breathing rhythm so that the mind can be pacified?
From this insight, many pranayamas came to be.
A simple evidence - if you watch your breath
or become aware of your breath, the breath slows down.*

~ Sri M, The Satsung Foundation

Human beings are complicated, this much is true. Ironically, we already have a solution to easing burdens and challenges to handle life's twists and turns, if we only take a moment to pause, reflect and breathe.

For me, the value of taking this moment came experientially, a distillation of the years of study and practice of asana (postures), pranayama (breath control), massage therapy, and energy work.

My first introduction to breathing as a "thing" occurred in yoga classes in the late 70s. A good friend took me to a yoga class, and a new world opened. It was a huge change for a fast-moving, speaking, thinking high school teacher (my second career) who didn't comprehend what being responsible for me really meant. I had lived just enough life to know there was something the ancient healing arts offered that I hadn't encountered anywhere else.

"Sit still and be quiet" was a totally new concept! I often squirmed like a child in kindergarten, antsy to go outside and play. Except as an adult, it involved writing lesson plans and grading papers. Learning some crazy positions for my body, including wiggling my toes, gradually got my undivided attention. We laughed regularly even as we were challenged. This evolved into studying a proper way to sit, stand, bend, twist, and invert (asanas) and controlled breathing patterns (pranayama). As running and gym workouts didn't interest me, this method of movement, breathing, and focus was attractive to my mind and body, and a daily practice quite readily came into being.

During a two-week yoga immersion on the Greek island of Lesvos, both asana and pranayama became a way of living, not just something to do with my physical body. The fresh, clean air and the soothing surf sounds of the Aegean Sea personified the themes of quietude and effortlessness, which international teachers Angela Farmer and Victor Von Kooten exemplified. For twists, Victor would say, "Feel your body move as if slowly spiraling out of the shell; be more playful." For breathing, Angela would say, "Inhalation and exhalation happen, like connecting with the beloved."

The richness of the island experience led to an event of heightened connection to the divine on the very last day after the last class. Angela and Victor led 35 men and women into a deep meditation. During it, I envisioned a young woman in a flowing white dress with the sweetest smile. She had a message for me to give to the class. This was startling, as I had never had such an experience and was very hesitant, wondering if I had the nerve to speak as directed. Yet I did.

After class, I went to Angela, speechless yet wanting to know what she thought about what had just happened. She knew without my asking. Her quiet, kind eyes embraced me, and she asked, "Who do you think that was?" I gasped, waited, and said, "That was me, wasn't it?" And she knowingly and softly nodded.

To this day, I don't recollect the words I was given to share. However, the divine connection has remained tangible and alive through every single breath. The messages flow with the breath through words, touch, and presence throughout the most wise gift of all, the body.

After that early experience, the breath became my vehicle for feeling mothered, a coming home. I observed my own patterns. Inhalations of surprise, delight, startledness, fright, effort. Exhalations of relief, awe, laughter, speech, relaxation. Holding breaths when feeling uncertain, frustrated, challenged, labored, and focused. So much affected how I breathed and when I breathed from movements, organs, emotions, thoughts, and yet when quieted, a balance and ease emanated and pervaded.

Within a short time, my world changed dramatically when I opened a healing center as a first-time business owner, yoga teacher, and massage therapist.

During one evening yoga class, a student came rushing into the room short of breath, fraught by her lateness due to car problems and embarrassment for disturbing the class. She grew more upset when I quietly welcomed her to join us where we were in an easy seated position. She couldn't settle down even though that was what she wanted most. I invited the whole class to join her in standing and begin to take longer, slower inhalations and exhalations and then to remain quiet with an easy breath. She was able to settle into an easier attitude. Everyone began to smile, and we talked about how we can easily and quickly change with breath focus.

Steadily, I gravitated to more moments of silky-smooth breathing to counter the increasing responsibilities, stresses, and time demands. I already had daily 30-90-minute asana and pranayama practices and had begun a twice-a-day seated meditation practice—sitting quietly, being with my breath, with no control, led to sensations as if listening to the sweetness of the strings of a symphony orchestra. It was a feeling of belonging and bliss that I could define but never experienced.

In the middle of a busy day, I sometimes sneaked five minutes in an empty massage room or even sat in the car for a few moments before starting it. Those moments were like a frozen stream melting, beginning to gurgle in the warm spring sunshine.

Fast forward: After selling the Center, space rentals and house calls became the norm, with fewer responsibilities and more time for my practices. Then, a long visit from Covid fatigue affected everything. I hit the proverbial brick wall! No practices, schedules, students, clients, meetings, writing, lectures, travel—total external non-activity.

The Being Breath was born out of my Covid fatigue experience. This is one time I'm so glad that my *modus operandi* this lifetime has been to see the positive in everything.

At the start, the very breath of me felt robbed by the phenomenon that changed our world. One day, I awoke feeling achy, feverish, and fatigued. The fatigue lasted an entire year. Early on, the amount of energy required to walk from my bedroom to the kitchen, read, make decisions or choices, listen to music, or talk on the phone exhausted me. It was as if the thinking mind and emotional body went on vacation! My physical and spirit energy bodies were in charge of healing.

With lots of time in bed or in a reclining chair, being with my breathing was my only solace. It was sometimes steady and sometimes not, yet these rhythms still provided a base—a coming home. Even in illness, a sense of connecting to the very basic rhythm of life was simple and effortless.

Easy breathing, natural breathing has a profundity. The inhaling: receiving the air around me. The pausing: processing this intake, penetrating and transforming the oxygen for the energy to live and heal. The exhaling: what isn't needed returning to the planet. The pausing: a shift into restfulness and deep dives into feeling divinely connected. It all just happened!

Healing had been happening as well—a natural inter- and intra-connectedness rhythm of the body. There was nothing I could do or control. It was just magic: innate intelligence and wisdom.

Now healthy, I sometimes forget when there's one more email to respond to before sleep, there's a piece of dark chocolate that calls my name, or a client who calls in pain. The usual signs of my forgetting are compromised elimination, strained breathing, frustration, forgetfulness, and bass fiddle strings for neck muscles with walnuts for the trapezius!

Fortunately, "sit still and be quiet" and "pay attention to your breath" soften these labored physical, mental, and emotional reactions. Even though they still re-appear occasionally, I no longer berate them. They're now my messengers to remember to inhale, pause, and exhale, pause, so I can breathe easily and return home to remember the magic.

The natural breathing process, which I call "Being Breath," keeps us on a steady course: receiving, experiencing, and returning to the mother. It is the ballast for sustaining, even more so, cultivating all the other rhythms of daily living. The Being Breath is the mother of all our bodies' natural physical, mental, emotional, and spiritual rhythms. As complicated human beings with a multitude of natural rhythms, one for each organ and action, even each word, we have the capacity to be joyously alive.

We each have been gifted the rhythm of breathing, from the first breath to the last. No one is different or left out of this divine design. No special equipment, clothes, or location is required. Let's get you started cultivating familiarity and friendliness with what you already have and will always have within you: the ability to come home to yourself.

THE TOOL

Being Breath is the expression of the innate intelligence of the body. Its easy rhythm is effortless effort: muscles must contract and release, nerve endings communicate to and from the brain, and chemistry is changed within organs, with no extra effort needed to make these changes. When you experience forced breathing, a raggedness, or shallowness during your day, it's your body's way of talking to you, saying change something! Here is an easy start for feeling more comfortable at home in your own body and making choices for ease and simplicity.

SETTING - TIME AND PLACE

When and where we place ourselves affects not only our thinking but also our breathing. Breath is our first guide to letting us know if we feel safe.

- Choose a time in your day dedicated to just you (even three minutes is enough to start). This is when you know there will be no outside demands from family, friends, work, etc. Sometimes, first thing in the morning, last thing in the evening, or even in the middle of the day.

- Choose a location that is quieter than not, with few to no electronic devices turned on and no people or animals. Comfortable clothes, a chair, and temperature are encouraged.

- Sometimes, sitting in the car before turning it on or after turning it off is even suitable. Note: not while driving!

BODY DETAILS FOR BEING BREATH

STRUCTURE AND ALIGNMENT

Start noticing from bottom to top, from feet to head. Sit in a comfortable chair with feet on the floor, bent knees aligning over ankles, buttocks moved to the back of chair seat supported by the chair back, front spine elongating, shoulder blades descending, palms comfortably resting on thighs, head and eyes leveling. Aligning your bone structure over joints immediately gives the body a sense of balance, strength, and ease.

Another way to say this is the back body skin, flesh, and bones descend as the front body's spine, rib cage, sternum, and collar bones ascend.

If this is uncomfortable, you may need support in one or more areas. A different chair could do the trick. Or add the support of pillows, blankets, blocks, etc. (get creative). The areas where you might need support include:

- under your feet (the chair is too short for your feet to touch the floor comfortably)

- under your hips and thighs (the chair is too short for the length of your legs)

- behind your sacrum (one of the simplest ways to lengthen the spine)

- behind your head (even with your spine elongated, the neck may curve forward and not rest over the shoulder girdle).

ROOTING

Imagination often plays a big part when inviting the body to change. It is a normal part of the mind's functions yet has no harsh demands on the body. This rooting step starts with imagining a tree growing roots (as in an oak tree, not a palm), with many long, sinewy roots reaching out from the following areas.

Feet: toes, ball mounts, sides of feet, and heel mounts.

Pelvis: two sitting bones and tailbone.

Shoulder blades points

All these places are rooting toward the pelvis, toward the feet, and the planet. Thus, as mentioned above, the back body feels like it is descending. All areas of rooting happen simultaneously and effortlessly.

ROUNDNESS OF BREATHING ANATOMY

The entire body is rounded everywhere, much like nature's innate design. As the back body descends and the front spine lengthens, the chest and head bones and organs of breathing are rounded, all enhanced with this chosen alignment. The diaphragm is asymmetrical and shaped like a mushroom cap, rounded; twelve ribs are rounded, including the top ribs under the curved collar bones; two lungs are cone-shaped round; the trachea is a round tube connecting the lungs to the nostrils through the throat. All are rounded, effortlessly.

This is in opposition to the new teaching norm of pushing out the abdomen on the inhalation. Problems with this practice include 1) there are no breathing organs in the abdomen, 2) the abdominal area is hardened as it's pushed forward, and 3) the effort of forced breathing strains the chest and throat. This is antithetical to the peaceful state of Being Breath.

FOUR PARTS OF NATURAL, SILKY-SMOOTH BREATHING: INHALATION, PAUSE SPACE, EXHALATION, PAUSE SPACE

- Feel, sensing your inhalation and the exhalation. If this is challenging, imagine it happening, as it must be to be alive.

• Notice three aspects of the inhalation: the length, the rhythm, and the effort or effortlessness. Then, notice the same for the exhalation. None of this is for right versus wrong evaluation, but to determine how it is, a reference point of what's happening as you begin this awareness practice. Take your time. It may be a moment or two before discerning these patterns of your natural flow, which happens without effort or external control.

• Next, observe the two pause spaces: the place where a breath isn't an inhale before it becomes an exhale, and a second place where the breath isn't an exhale before it becomes an inhale. Each has its own length and effortlessness. Stay with this long enough to identify these spaces.

• Now, continue observing all four parts, from inhalation to pause space to exhalation to pause space. When enough is enough, return to just the Being Breath flow, without sensing patterns.

• Three minutes is a good length to start practicing this observation. In the beginning, setting a timer can help ease timing concerns. Sometimes, you may not observe all the above steps. Sometimes, you may fall asleep. Building awareness takes time and practice.

• Whatever you experience is an effective practice of awareness; there are no goals to meet. Interestingly, the longer you stay quietly involved with this natural flow, the shift to noticing will often change the rhythm and pattern. Again, just observe, sense. This is also very natural and normal.

Initially, this may seem like a very simple and unfruitful practice. However, sensations of harmony, happiness, and balance are real. Laughter and love come readily; you may find yourself guffawing out loud! With the daily demands on all aspects of living in the now, an increased external demand has changed the definition of natural and normal. Holding breath, tense breathing, and unawareness of breathing are natural but not normal. They've only become more and more familiar. Living really does happen one breath at a time.

For experienced practitioners, this Being Breath pattern is beneficial to repeat regularly. We all tend to stay in a practiced breath pattern and neglect the natural flow.

Welcome to the first steps of cultivating your natural life rhythm through breath awareness, one breath at a time.

I look forward to hearing about your experiences with the Being Breath. Know there are many more practices, including more controls and yoga props. I'll be happy to answer your questions or guide you on Zoom (or in person). Contact me directly at yoginikandy62@gmail.com.

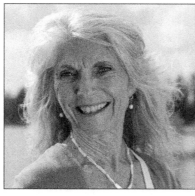

Kandy Taylor Love, PhD, CIYT, LMT, Child of the Divine

For more than 45 years, Kandy's eclectic skill set and continuing study and practice have made her an inspirational and progressive yoga teacher, mentor, and bodyworker.

As a healer, she blends the natural health practices of yoga, massage therapies, and meditation in the clinical, classroom (in person and on Zoom), and corporate settings. Kandy holds herself as a springboard for students and clients to rediscover the playful, powerful, and peaceful aspects of themselves.

More specifically, her toolkit includes principles of yoga in the Iyengar style, breathwork, and massage techniques, including craniosacral therapy, whole-body healing based on Healing from the Core® and Integrated Awareness®. The development of daily practices for living in harmony is key.

LoveWorks is her business, one-on-one custom-designed healing sessions, which include drawing from the toolkit, listening, holding containers, and simply being compassionate and present.

Kandy has fun with her name, and yes, "Love" is her given name. Not only did her loving parents give her this sometimes fun and sometimes problematic challenge from birth, but they also instilled the joy of being in nature, traveling, continuing learning, and being of service.

This blessed upbringing led to two heart-centered manifestations: owning and operating a healing center for 25 years and traveling to teach, touch, and study in seven countries and many US states.

Her desire to touch more lives has led to authoring two collaborative books, co-producing Carpel Tunnel Coaching (an online healing program), and recording five albums on yoga and meditation (three with Amazon's #1 recommended *Gulf Coast Meditations*).

Kandy's vision is a world where everyone feels comfortable, beautiful, and magical in their own skin.

To enhance your journey with a video version of The Being Breath, go to www.becauseloveworks.com. For a free consult, contact her directly at yoginikandy62@gmail.com or visit facebook.com/kandy.t.love

CHAPTER 12

BREAKING THE ANCESTRAL CYCLE

USING EFT TO HEAL EMOTIONAL EATING FROM GENERATIONAL WOUNDS

Denise Flood

MY STORY

"Your brother is dead." In that instant, I felt myself leave my body.

Looking down, I saw myself standing dumbfounded.

"I want to see him."

"No, you don't. He's been in a car accident."

My parents sat in shock in the grieving room, set aside for bad news, in the corner of the Emergency Room, and I was asked to leave the room when the doctor came in. Alone, I stepped outside.

The nurse said, "Don't cry. You have to be strong for your parents."

The neighbor said, "Don't cry. You have to be strong for your parents."

And later, teachers said, "Don't cry. You have to be strong for your parents."

The priest said, "Don't cry. You have to be strong for your parents."

The nuns said, "Don't cry. You have to be strong for your parents."

My parents asked what was wrong with me. "Don't you care? Didn't you love your brother?"

The next morning, I awoke. *If I don't open my eyes, it will all be just a horrible nightmare. . .don't move. . .stay still and it will be undone.* I desperately grasp onto the hope that by refusing to acknowledge it, I can rewrite the outcome and bring him back to life. I pretended until I heard the sobs. I came downstairs to see my father on his knees, clinging to the windowsill. Bawling, I'd never seen him cry before. The sound tore through me, wiping away all hope. I walked dully into the heavy sorrow that permeated the room.

People began to arrive, and the meticulous planning commenced, orchestrating each detail as anticipation hung in the air like a heavy curtain. First, the viewing. I was horrified to see his corpse laid out, to have people come with their platitudes, thickened the atmosphere. A storm raged within me, *shut the fuck up!* I screamed inside my head. *You don't understand, it's not God's Will. How the Hell would you know?* echoed in my head as I nodded and numbly shook hands and accepted hugs. Looking composed and dutifully sorrowful on the outside.

After the funeral, we gathered at home. That's when I heard it first.

"It's too bad it had to be Michael," and murmurs of agreement. My fifteen-year-old self heard, "It should have been Denise." My grandmother's words shattered my heart the most.

The pain seared my soul. This moment was forever frozen in time and space; my gut clenched. Even in his death, I was judged as unworthy. I'd never be good enough.

I'll never be my brother.

I'll never be a man.

I'll never be worthy of carrying the family name.

His death was unexpected—just 17. At his birth, my mother's parents tried to pay my dad to change Michael's last name to carry on their legacy. "Not our firstborn," replied my father.

Two years later, I was born—already a disappointment to them (a girl). Born into the lesser. Raised as the reason we have sin and temptation in the world.

Accepting that the actions of others brought pain and shame was exalted as sacrifice and suffering for proof of how we loved Christ. It never set right inside me watching my mother lessen herself to be the dutiful wife.

My mother worked before she met my father. After they married, he insisted she stop working. Thus, I became the child of a frustrated woman. The only outlet allowed her was us, to keep house, and cook.

She cooked and presented each dinner with a tangible neediness. Full table settings for every meal. I, the girl, had the dishes and cleaned up. Every meal. Every day.

Resentment burned in me like a wildfire. I began to hate eating and everything about the kitchen. That's when the battles raged at the dinner table. Refusing to eat, I sat at my place. My father snarled, "You'll eat what's on your plate." I sat in silence. The air hit me first, then the slap that flung me onto the floor. I struggled to sit up. Then, he grabbed me by the hair, lifted me, and smashed my face into the plate of spaghetti. Sauce and noodles smeared all over my face. And, with a grunt of effort, he aggressively dragged me to the basement door. "You will not defy me." He flung the door open, kicked me through, and I tumbled down the stairs. In tears, I picked myself up defiantly and wiped my face off with his pristine white sailcloth, then snuck out the basement door. Battle lines drawn.

You'd think I could escape in school—no! My school was an extension of frustrated women (yes, nuns) in a small backwater town, bent on beating the devil out of us and making sure we knew in no uncertain terms that there were starving children in Africa who'd love to have our lunch. God forbid you mouth off and tell them you'd like to send it to them or try to hide the liver in your milk carton.

They'd send it home with you, and yes, my parents would serve it to me for dinner. And if I still refused, it was saved for breakfast, lunch, then dinner. If I were lucky, they'd leave the room long enough for me to feed it to the dog.

"Why can't you be more like your brother?" was the catchphrase of my childhood.

With his death, all of that came crashing down. I remained split, one part dutiful daughter, the other raging and confused. Over and over, I heard, "It was God's will." I questioned: *God's Will. What the fuck did that mean?* For me, it meant nothing mattered. No plans, no future. No hopes and dreams. It could all be stripped away at any moment.

And since I absorbed the message that everyone wished it was me who died, I threw myself at life as hard as I could, numbing myself with food, stuffing it down like I did my sorrow and confusion. Overeating, bloated, and alone.

I began drinking—drinking to oblivion and smoking pot to avoid feeling or talking to anyone. When I wasn't stoned (or drunk), I'd pretend I was so everyone left me alone.

No one confronted me, including teachers, friends, neighbors, or parents. No one wanted to talk about death. There were no school counselors. Psychiatrists were only for "crazy people" who belonged in the mental ward. And through all this, I still went home and pretended to be the dutiful child who tried to be both daughter and son.

I graduated high school and walked across that stage drunk. Then, I went to college, wasting four years away wallowing in self-abuse and hurting many along the way, and yes, I graduated drunk.

I knew that if I was to survive, I needed to leave that town, so I took the first opportunity to move to Florida in 1982. I felt like I could reinvent myself. Within a month, I discovered the "hippie farmers market" in Coconut Grove. My eyes opened to life beyond the confines of my Catholic upbringing. There were crystals, singing bowls, yoga, chanting, and organic foods. Slowly, my soul felt more like a part of my physical body.

I joined a spiritual belly dance troupe focused on the dance's traditional death and rebirth aspects. My body became less shameful step by step and movement by movement.

As I began nourishing myself on more than the physical level, I discovered how much there was to healing. For quite a few years, I was a sort of therapy junkie, meaning I learned as many different healing techniques as I could find. I moved into light body work and magnified healing from Reiki to Silva Mind Control. I thrived in new, healthier communities, my life opened, and my body became a place of release and healing.

I discovered flower essences and essential oils and was introduced to the world of frequency healing. Not every day was my best day; I learned about layers of healing and the onion concept of peeling back layers as they reveal. I slowly learned to love and trust a man who would become my husband and our daughter's father after five years of friendship. That's when I made even more soul-searching changes. Perhaps it's true for you that you'll make changes for a loved one that you wouldn't make for yourself as quickly.

I wanted my daughter to have a much different childhood than mine. I wanted her to feel loved and cherished from womb to birth (and beyond). I didn't want to expose her to anything that didn't validate that she was, above all else, a beloved soul.

It was at this time I discovered tapping. I'd become an early reading specialist for a small private school, and they sent me for training in Cross Brain Therapies and tapping/Emotional Freedom Technique (EFT) to help children reduce fear and stress around reading, testing, and learning new things. The results in the classroom astounded me, and as I took additional training, I saw the value in tapping with adults and clearing trauma, starting with my own.

Tapping is a way of gently bringing up things blocking us, harming us, and/or releasing habits that do not serve us. It's a way of clearing them gently and tapping into those higher vibrations, dreams, and aspirations we want to manifest in this world.

I compare it to how you'd clean your floors. You'd want to sweep your floors and get in the corners and the crevices before you wipe them down. Then you'd mop and clean those floors before you polish them.

For years, I called myself a child of trauma. Have I completely healed? No. I'm still on and of this Earth.

My father's anger and my mother's submission surface unexpectedly to this day.

Though I swore I wouldn't be my mother's daughter, in many ways, I am.

Though I swore I would never strike out in anger like my father, I have. I'm in my 60s, and still, moments of triggered rage engulf me.

Only now, though much trauma and self-discovery work, have I been able to diffuse without harm to self or others. And I'd like to offer this healing work to you.

THE TOOL

As we embark on this journey together, I invite you to give yourself permission to breathe deeply and fully. Allow yourself the time and space to be gentle, embracing each moment with kindness and understanding. Before we begin, grab a glass of water to sip on. For releasing and healing work, hydration is key. Have a pen and paper handy, ready to jot down any insights or reflections that arise along the way. After the first round of tapping, take a moment to go inward and self-assess. Notice the shifts within you and allow yourself to adjust gently, honoring the beautiful journey of self-discovery and growth that lies ahead. Let's tap into the power of healing together!

Part 1: Healing Generational Wounds

1. Find a quiet and comfortable space to focus on yourself without distractions. Take a few deep breaths, allowing yourself to relax and release any tension you may be holding onto. Acknowledge that you're part of a lineage with its own set of experiences and traumas that may have been passed down through generations.

2. Tap gently on the side of your hand or karate chop point (right under your pinky finger) while repeating the following affirmation three times: "Even though I carry wounds from past generations, I choose to heal and break free from their hold on me."

3. Tap on the following acupressure points while acknowledging out loud or in your mind any inherited pain or patterns, stating out loud or in your mind:

- Eyebrow: "I feel the weight of generational wounds."
- Side of the eye: "These patterns that have been passed down."
- Under the eye: "The pain that echoes through my family history."
- Under the nose: "Even though it's not mine, I've felt its impact."
- Chin: "I release the burdens that are not mine to carry."
- Collarbone: "I break the cycle of suffering and create a new legacy of healing."
- Under the arm: "I choose love and forgiveness over resentment and pain."
- Top of the head: "I am liberated from the past and embrace my path of healing and growth."

4. Take another deep breath and tune into your emotions and sensations. Notice any shifts in your perception or feelings of lightness and relief. Repeat the tapping process if there are still lingering emotions until you feel a sense of release and renewal.

Part 2: Clearing Emotional Eating

1. Continue in your comfortable space, taking a few more deep breaths to center yourself.

2. Tap gently on the side of your hand or karate chop point while repeating the following affirmation three times: "Even though I have used food to cope with my emotions, I deeply and completely love and accept myself."

3. Tap on the following acupressure points while stating out loud or in your mind any feelings or thoughts related to emotional eating:

- Eyebrow: "This urge to eat when I'm not hungry."
- Side of the eye: "These emotions that seem to control me."
- Under the eye: "The comfort I seek in food."
- Under the nose: "Even though food has been my escape, I choose to find healthier ways to cope."
- Chin: "I release the need to use food to numb my emotions."

- Collarbone: "I honor my body's true needs and nourish it with love."
- Under the arm: "I forgive myself for past patterns and embrace positive changes."
- Top of the head: "I am in control of my choices, and I choose health and balance."

4. Take a deep breath and assess how you feel. Notice any shifts in your emotions or sensations in your body. Repeat the tapping process if lingering emotions remain until you feel a sense of calm and empowerment.

Part 3: Integration and Empowerment

1. Take a moment to reflect on the journey you've just taken through tapping. Acknowledge the strength and courage it took to confront these deep-seated issues and commit to your well-being.

2. Tap gently on your heart center while affirming three times: "I am worthy of love, healing, and transformation."

3. Visualize yourself living a life free from the weight of generational wounds and emotional eating. See yourself making empowered choices, nourishing your body and soul with love and compassion.

4. Take a final deep breath, feeling gratitude for the healing journey you've embarked upon. Carry this sense of empowerment with you as you step forward into a brighter, more fulfilling future.

Remember, tapping is a powerful tool. It's essential to be patient and compassionate with yourself as you navigate these deep emotional waters. Allow yourself to seek additional support as needed, and know that healing is always possible with time, effort, and self-love.

Gift: Exclusive video download, Tapping to Heal Generational Wounds and Emotional Eating https://deniseflood.com/HVW

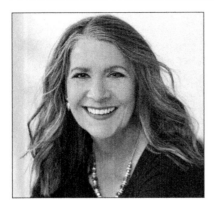

Denise Flood: Empowering Transformations through Energy Work

Denise Flood, a seasoned practitioner with over 35 years of experience in energy work, offers a unique self-care program blending many techniques for profound transformation and healing. Inspired by her journey through life's challenges, Denise provides individuals with an extraordinary opportunity for holistic well-being and self-discovery.

Professional Journey and Expertise

Throughout her career, Denise immersed herself in studying healing energy, integrating aromatherapy, meditation, Light Body Healing, Reiki, and EFT into her practice. Her intuitive understanding of clients' needs allows her to create a nurturing environment where individuals unlock their true potential.

Denise's signature program focuses on personalized tapping meditation scripts, tailored to address individual challenges and goals. Participants embark on a holistic journey of self-discovery, emerging with enhanced well-being and a profound connection to their authentic selves.

Why Partner with Denise Flood?

Denise offers more than a program; she provides a pathway to lasting change and transformation. Her expertise and genuine passion for helping others make her a trusted guide toward holistic well-being. Through this transformative practice, participants are guided to explore the depths of their consciousness, releasing emotional blockages and aligning with their highest potential.

Referrals

"Denise Flood's voice brings me instant peace and calm. Her expertise has been an invaluable asset to our family." ~Tatianna M.

"Tapping with Denise Flood has been insightful for many issues. She not only helped me begin to feel safe, she created short tapping meditations I can play anytime." ~Debi C.

Seize the Moment

The opportunity for Divine Transformation awaits. Embark on a transformative journey with Denise Flood today. Contact her to begin your path toward profound healing, empowerment, and self-discovery. This is your moment for lasting change—seize it now and step into the vibrant, authentic life you deserve.

Connect with Denise today:

https://deniseflood.com/

https://tinyurl.com/immerseyourselfyoutube

https://www.facebook.com/changeyourfrequencychangeyourlife

CHAPTER 13

THE GIFT OF LIGHT LANGUAGE

USING YOUR VOICE TO HEAL YOUR LIFE

Caroline Mary

"And the truth will set you free."

~ John 8.32

MY STORY

Here we go; it's coming out again. Light language. The sound of my soul, and one of my favorite things in the world. But does it have to burst out like this?

"Ma Koi, danay-sha, moi kash kamoi dinoi-ya sha-kowa moi-yaka."

It pours out of me as I watch the lady dressed in colorful, flowing clothes glide around the crystal shop I'm minding for a friend. Her long hair flutters as she moves in and out of the trailing scarves and decorations hanging throughout the shop.

I hope she's alright with this. It feels alright. It must be alright.

"Ka-ma koia kisha noi, throia cha kashoi-a," I continue, sharing the light language bursting through me.

She turns towards me and smiles.

"Sayaaaa moka la, shaaa moi ka," she replies a little bashfully in her own light language.

Oh my God! She gets it!

"What are we speaking?" she asks as she moves closer to the counter I'm sitting behind.

"Light language! It's from the stars: it's our soul speak!" I blurt out.

"Ahh, I see," she says, smiling even wider. "It's incredible. I spoke this as a child, but I've always hidden it from other people."

She's glowing and continues sharing, "Do you know something? I've just received an answer. I've been pondering about something, and I know the answer, clear as day."

I love it! I love the clarity that comes after speaking light language. It's just incredible.

Years later, Sarah is a dear friend, and we enjoy speaking in light language while weaving around each other on a dance floor. To this day, Sarah never lets me forget the time we shared light language; her life changed forever.

The time her voice was liberated, and she received the clarity she needed just like I do.

Light language is a passion of mine because of the alignment that happens as we speak it. It comes straight from our hearts, so many of us can access these languages from our soul memory. When we activate them, we gain a greater connection to our soul's wisdom and a feeling of coming home.

I didn't always speak light language, though. In fact, at times in my life, I could barely speak. I died of embarrassment just thinking about saying my name out loud, and sometimes, I mumbled it, having to repeat it again and again to people.

I needed to know why I struggled like this, so I asked my mother what I was like as a child and whether I spoke to people back then.

"You were usually well-behaved. Sometimes you'd hide behind your dad, but only when you were very little," she replied. Nothing stood out for her as unusual, especially not about my speech.

I asked myself: *Why did I seem normal as a child and then struggle to speak to people later? Was I well-behaved, or was I following the lead of people around me?*

It didn't make sense, and I still didn't understand why my voice would fail or change. One minute I was talking, and the next, I was silent. Stunned and frozen, words would fail to appear, and it was embarrassing, especially if you couldn't reply when asked a question.

Digging into memories as I began my healing journey, I remembered I didn't speak light language as a kid like Sarah, but I used to squeal. *And wow, did I squeal! No problem making sounds back then.*

I recall running around the garden with the sunshine warming our skin and the hum of bees in the air. Water drops cooled us and twinkled in the sunlight as we dodged in and out of the arc of the water sprinkler. Joy was in the air, and our school holidays were just around the corner.

"Eeeeh! Weee! Eeeeh!" I'm squealing with joy as I fly around, acting like an airplane, chasing my friend around her garden.

"Yaaaaaaaaaaaaaaaaa! Eeeeeeee—"

"Stop that now! Can't you keep it quiet!?" shouts a neighbor over the fence, crushing our joy. We're silenced to the core, and my joyful energy plummets. I shrink into myself, and not long after, Mum picks me up, and we walk home in silence. I'm stunned the rest of the evening, my voice squashed for years to come.

After this memory surfaced, more memories came to light when adults shushed us young ones—teachers, relatives, and neighbors who didn't realize the effects they'd have later on. "Don't be so silly!" they'd say, or "Keep it quiet!"

Despite this suppression of my voice, I found other ways to express myself in my teenage years, and it feels like a soul gift to have overcome the challenge of suppression in this way. Playing in orchestras, choirs, and the school jazz band, I loved feeling music flowing through me and hearing it all around. It was a gift of childhood in that respect, and my parents supported me in making the most out of my musicianship.

Later on, however, leaving school without an instrument to hand, I barely said a word. I went out alone, finding somewhere I could dance, eyes closed and moving freely. I expressed myself in a way I couldn't when I was with people.

Regular weekends of ecstatic dancing led to intense phases of awakening in my 20s.

Flowing with energy, I felt alive and inspired. At times, reams of information flooded my mind with visions of the future where people lived for longer and mostly lived on light, eating only minimal natural foods. These people existed in harmony with each other and nature, and the feelings of hope filled me. *A hope I'd lost growing up in the 80s, I realized.*

It felt like ancient wisdom was moving through me, and I sensed the energy of spirits around me, offering comfort in this strange yet somehow familiar time in my life. I spent days in meditation, receiving an understanding of my life and the world around me.

As the intensity of these awakenings ebbed away and I started to integrate back into life, I felt alone and shut down again. The people around me didn't seem to see the world as I did. I pushed these experiences to the back of my mind and got on with life, plodding on with mundane jobs, looking forward to the weekend when I'd be free on the dance floor.

Despite pushing these visions away, a seed was planted. I felt confused, having tasted the future without clarity about my part in it or how humanity would ever get there. I'd all but given up hope until I went traveling in my early 30s.

During these travels, I met spiritual, open-minded people, and it became clear I wasn't alone in my experiences. Many had similar visions, heard voices of guides and loved ones from the other side, and received information through intuition. I just hadn't met them before.

Near the end of this trip, I found myself in a ceremony that changed my life. We were at a small healing festival and gathered inside a teepee. A Romanian shaman was calling in healing for the group, and some of the people started to lie down to receive healing while others sat up, holding space for their friends. After a while, I found myself standing up and chanting. Sounds were coming out of me that I'd never made before. It felt so good!

Energy was moving through me, and my body was swaying as the sound continued to come through me. Long drones and strange languages poured out, and the shaman looked on as though he knew what was happening.

Though this was a surprise, it felt right, and I felt at home channeling these sounds. It felt like my soul had come alive, and I knew exactly what to do at the perfect time. It seemed familiar and reminded me of the awakenings I experienced in my 20s.

Later in this ceremony, I felt a strong urge to cut my dreadlocks and shave my head; it was a new beginning. After shedding my hair, I started shedding other things connecting me to my old life: my clothes, craft materials, and more. Slowly but surely, my belongings left my life.

As this shedding continued, I returned from my travels, not knowing where life would take me. I moved to a new city, and a new life seemed to unfold. I attended Ecstatic Awakening Dance training, which profoundly changed my life. I met a dear soul sister whose psychic gifts and worldview permitted me to explore my experiences without fear.

She spoke an other-worldly language, too, and it seemed completely normal for her. "It's my star language, Caroline, there's nothing weird about it," was her down-to-earth explanation. "People call it light language," she confirmed.

Little did I know how light language would continue to show up in my life when I was asked to channel healing for a Peruvian shaman a few months later. Light language streamed through me as I placed my hands on the gentle older man lying by my side. I felt at home again, and another seed was planted.

Over the next few years, I continued to give away or sell my belongings, and the biggest challenge was letting go of my instruments: djembes, my dear saxophone, oboe, flute, clarinet, guitars, CDJs, shakers, singing bowls, and more were sold or given away.

One by one, they all went, and my heart broke every time another instrument left with its new owner. My flat became emptier than ever. *What on Earth am I doing? Why do I have to give all this up? It better be worth it cos this sucks.*

What was the gift of all the releasing?

Light language. *And healing. So much healing.*

Without the trappings of my former life, there was space, and I met teachers, healers, guides, and friends who assisted me in coming home to myself and ever more express my truth. My awakening experiences became normal, and my life changed beyond recognition. I found the self buried beneath the instruments, suppression, hippy clothes, and the dreadlocks. I came home.

As a published author, I hold space for others through coaching and workshops, and I love sharing my insights through social media and writing projects. I'm able to speak my truth and, in doing so, live my truth.

Light language is one of my go-to offerings to help others clear their throat chakra and share their truth. It can assist people in accessing their innate healing capacity and soul wisdom, and it's a tangible healing gift to share with others.

You might think if you speak in light language, "People won't understand me," however, they will *inner*-stand you. They will *feel* the energy with their body rather than *understand* with their mind.

They, like you, will feel the joy and clarity light language brings due to the high vibrational energy we transmit when we speak it. It heals us, filling us with light from our higher self as we allow ourselves to be conduits of these beautiful light languages.

I pondered the significance of light language when I sat in one of my favorite nature spots and spoke to guides about this project. One of so many healing tools we can access right now, I asked them, "Why is it so important? Why am I sharing this?"

It's your truth, and the truth will set you free, came the answer.

I knew he didn't mean me but humanity as a family. Speaking our truth in our birth language or our soul language, *light language,* meant we were aligning with our truth, which was our liberation.

In this time where we can read about breatharians (people who live on light), long lives, and energy healing, it seems like my vision of a distant future is coming ever closer, and sharing light language with you is part of that future unfolding.

We are creating that future by speaking our truth, by living our truth.

THE TOOL

USING YOUR VOICE TO HEAL YOUR LIFE

STEP 1 - SOUND IT OUT

Take a few moments to sound out your feelings using anything but words.

Start with an "Ahh" and move into different sounds, such as ooh, ahh, laa, maa, when you're ready and lose yourself in the moment. This is an ecstatic dance for your voice.

It can be challenging, I know, so it can help to know you're probably going to sound silly, so be ok with sounding silly! Try not to censor any sounds coming out.

Right now, be silly, sound silly, look silly, and enjoy making different noises and stretching your mouth and tongue! Open your mouth wide, stretch it, move it in ways you wouldn't normally, and see how it feels. Allow yourself to have fun with it, as I do when I'm working with a group.

The more you loosen up, the easier it will flow: you cannot think and speak light language like you cannot think and dance freely.

This practice is a great way to release attachment from our birth languages and get used to creating sounds without using words we're familiar with. Have fun!

STEP 2 - ACTIVATING YOUR LIGHT LANGUAGE

Visit: https://www.openlotusliving.com/the-gift-of-light-language. You'll hear me speaking in a few different light languages as I activate yours. You may want to listen a few times, and as you listen, join in as and when you can.

Allow yourself to receive the energy of the transmission, and when you're ready, express any sounds that want to come through you. It can help to imagine you are responding to me with your language, and we're having a conversation.

Don't try to copy me in this exercise, as your language may sound very different, with clicks, high pitches, low pitches, or something in the middle. You may also sound like a bird or feel like a dragon. It's all possible, and you aren't making it up. If it feels forced, let it go and start again.

A word of warning: once you start, I promise, you'll want to speak it wherever you are. You may well forget who you were as you open up to new callings in your life!

STEP 3 - SHARING YOUR GIFT OF LIGHT LANGUAGE

Choose a person or situation you'd like to bring healing to, and set the intention to bring healing for the highest good of all involved.

Let yourself express light language (or the sounds that have started to come to you) until the sounds naturally end. Please ask the person in question if you're bringing healing for them.

Light language can heal anything, and the energy it brings through you heals you at the same time. As you get used to it, you can use it wherever you are to clear your energy or bring healing to those around you.

STEP 4 - OPTIONAL WARM-UP TOOLS

1. Grounding: when we're working with energy, it can leave us feeling high and ungrounded, so you can use the following breath exercise to make sure you're feeling centered and grounded:

    Close your eyes and take an in-breath, and when you exhale, let your point of focus move down through your body and into the heart of Gaia. On your next breath, draw in the earth's energy and move your awareness up with the breath and out of the top of your head towards Source. As you breathe out, come back down with your attention and into Gaia again. Continue for a few breaths, then come back to simply observing your breath moving in and out. When you're ready, come back into the room.

2. Releasing: if you resist making sounds or light language, you may wish to explore what you believe about yourself and/or your abilities using EFT or journalling. Let go of any limitations and set yourself free!

3. Dancing: getting out of our heads helps us to free ourselves from our ego-brain and move into flow. Put on your favorite track and come into a flow state, then listen to the audio track on the link in Step 2 and enjoy.

It's my pleasure to share light language with the world, and I'm so happy to share it with you today. I hope you'll go over to the website, hear some for yourself, and see what unfolds for you as you do. If you'd like more inspiration, there are plenty of videos on the internet from others who speak light language, and it's my greatest wish it becomes as normal as hearing different earth languages.

May your voice and your joy flow with ease!

So much love to you.

Ka-moika, na shoya, ko-na maya koia, makoya shan a keyowa.

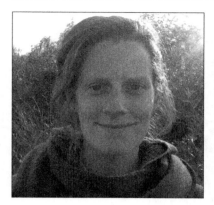

Caroline Mary is a co-author in another collaborative project, The Energy Healer's Oracle. She's a life coach, angelic healer, speaker of light language, and all-round ponderer of life. She's dedicated to assisting people to untie the knots of their inner realms so they can live a free and liberated life in alignment with their soul's calling.

Trained in various healing modalities, she's writing other healing modalities to assist in uplifting humanity as we move through these unprecedented times.

Caroline enjoys ecstatic dance or walking in the countryside in Wales. She loves to be near rivers, lakes, trees, and mountains, where she enjoys connecting to nature's spirits for wisdom and healing. She also loves cakes, chocolate, and period dramas.

Connect with Caroline:

Website: https://www.openlotusliving.com

Email: carolinemaryandrews@hotmail.com

Facebook: https://www.Facebook.com/CarolineMaryAndrews

CHAPTER 14

WHEN GLASS BREAKS

GETTING GROUNDED
IN CULINARY THERAPY

Joy E. Davis, LMSW

MY STORY

Cooking saved my life when my marriage fell apart.

Glancing at the clock, it's 2 a.m., and my eyes feel gritty like sandpaper. The 17-hour workday is hitting hard, and I am trying to be as quiet as possible so as not to wake my Husband. He knew we would be in late, just not this late. I dry off from the shower, wrap my damp hair in a towel and lotion, dress quickly to hit the couch and sleep for three hours before I need to be up and do it all over again. No one tells you when you are a chef for a small gourmet restaurant that you wear multiple hats, which include efficiency and workflow—every muscle hurts from moving the kitchen equipment around and unloading products from the supplier. I slowly turn off the light and open the bathroom door to avoid squeaking into the dark living room. I suck in my breath as my bare feet hit the cold slate tile and begin to tiptoe to the couch, which has become my bed of choice. I make it to the coffee table before he bursts open the bedroom door, backlit by the nightstand lamp from our bedroom.

I inwardly cringe. Unfortunately, the darkness does not hide the anger on his face. "What are you doing?! You're going to wake up everyone! Can't you tell people are sleeping?!"

I'm pretty sure you just did that by screaming.

"I'm trying to be quiet."

"Well, you're doing a piss poor job at it." He stalks toward me with evil in his eyes.

Here it comes. I try to shrink back because I know that look.

"You're the most selfish person I know; you cannot for one second consider others!" He stands before me so close that I can tell he brushed his teeth with Colgate. His eyes are bulging, and he's shaking with anger, placing mean hands on my upper arms and shaking me like a doll.

This angry display happened too many times to count. He continues to belittle and yell from what I can tell by his mouth still moving, though I retreat into myself to stop hearing the poison he is spewing. It's nothing new, just Tuesday. *Please go to bed and leave me alone.*

As he turns, he knocks whatever he left on the coffee table over, and it shatters on the slate floor all around my clean, bare feet. There's liquid running over like a waterfall with a sickening drip. "Look at what you made me do! How can you be so stupid to leave glass on the coffee table?! Clean it up! He marches back to the bedroom and slams the door.

Standing there surrounded by broken glass became a metaphor for my marriage. I had to walk on glass to get anywhere to clean up the mess; my feet bled, but I did it because I had no choice. That's the night I realized that twelve years and two therapists later, nothing could fix my broken and pulverized marriage. I am paralyzed, afraid to leave this comfortable dysfunction where I have died slowly over time, yet scared to stay because it will only get worse, completely suspended between the two choices of death or life. The internal conflict is overwhelming. I don't know how long I stood there weighing my choices as hot, bitter tears roll down my face. I've only considered him and everyone else. Not one person knows about this side of him or the personal Hell I lived in since our vows. I kept his secret because wives don't snitch on their husbands.

I automatically began to rationalize his unruly behavior. *It's my fault. I'm late*, and mid-thought, I realize I cannot do this anymore for him. As it is, I don't recognize myself or even like this version of myself. All I know is what he prefers and what role he wants me to play, especially for his church staff and choir students. I cannot be in this play anymore; I want out. *That's it. I cannot do this anymore.* I'm bleeding, and this is not the first time. I'm afraid if I don't leave him, I will die. I chose life. I chose the unknown and felt like God released me from my marriage and told me to fly.

"The moment you realize your life is not yours anymore, it can take a different shape and leap out of your hands. Your heart, in one breath, from one moment to the next, realizes you want something different, something more than this inauthentic hypocrisy you helped create and nourish. As soon as this realization happens, you cannot go back! That life is over; you need to bury it and grieve." (Davis, Joy, "Journal." 2009.)

My marriage was never together in the way most would think. There was never a honeymoon period or romantic butterflies or body worship, for that matter; it felt transactional, and this is what we do now. At the tender age of fourteen, I met my Husband, the youth leader and choral director at our church. He was twenty-one, and I thought, *this is it, no dating for me.* I told my parents I would marry him one day, and they probably thought I'd lost my mind—just a teen crush. I was dead serious. I thought I was getting my dream man and pursued him like air. I cultivated a deep friendship with him over long and short distances and endured his two long-term girlfriends until it was my turn. I know now that I did this all wrong. Pursuing a man is a dead end.

I'm curious if my confidence and determination in our relationship over ten years sealed the deal in his mind, and maybe he thought I would be a good wife. Who knows? I've long since accepted but I'll never know his whys. We dated for three years before he proposed at two a.m. on the phone and again in person. Not romantic, earth-shattering, or even planned out. He was the most remarkable patient person on the planet. I never saw him mad or upset during those first ten years, and at the time, I thought he knew, saw, and accepted me.

Fast forward three months into our marriage, I saw him mad for the first time. That first argument over something stupid was when I ran through the house to escape his rage and locked the bathroom door, hoping he would calm down and give me space. Instead, he broke the door down, message received, there was nowhere safe for me to escape from that moment on. Six months into our marriage, he sat me down through guilty tears and a boatload of foreboding, communicated he wasn't attracted to me and didn't know what to do, implying that I was a horrible human whom he no longer considered precious. I remember thinking my world was never going to be the same, and I took on all the blame. It didn't dare cross my mind that it could be anything other than my fault. My Husband never told me why he was not into me; he just said he wasn't. Entering the cave of shame, rejection, and self-loathing, I crawled in, made myself comfortable, and didn't resurface until culinary school. I went from the best shape of my life to the shell of a person abusing food for comfort. I was a version of me fit for public consumption, but not me in the authentic sense. *Ugh, I grew up to be his perfect woman. Who am I?* I had yet to explore.

All I knew was that he no longer desired me. That island was lonely. For me, that meant my marriage was over because I believed that you cannot manufacture desire or attraction. Other parts of love, yes, but not those things. We were barely intimate. Maybe, say, six times in twelve years, he said it was because he had already experienced things with ex-girlfriends; why did he need to continue with me? "Why are you such a whore, that you want more sex?" He was the only man I had. Sex became a tool he used to control. A rejection so complete that I ceased to exist. I no longer fit into my clothes or world and pretended to be okay. I was feeling trapped, lonely, rejected, and undesired. At this juncture in my marriage, this is when emotional, sexual, and physical abuse began. It lasted twelve years before I filed for divorce.

Culinary therapy was my lifeline. That first step outside of my brokenness to a new path, even before diving into personal trauma therapy. At the end of my marriage, I walked away, leaving all my material goods, financial security, house, and especially my wife role behind to cultivate a new life. One that I had little knowledge of how I would later heal or help others heal. I enrolled in culinary school at 34—the most challenging, most rewarding nine months of my life.

This pivotal time was when I chose myself over everyone else. It was a time of recognizing I had a voice and power that no one could take away. It was a time to step into God's purpose for my life, where no one made me—I made myself. No more people pleasing. It was about pleasing God and allowing myself to heal trauma responses and destructive thoughts about myself and marriage, learning my identity, and honing my culinary acumen. I developed core values and explored how I wanted to show up for the world as a victor, not a victim.

That's powerful when you've spent your entire life fitting in, not being a bother, being quiet, staying in good graces, not making a scene, or getting in trouble. I learned early on how to accommodate everyone's preferences. I didn't even know how to think or feel for myself.

Culinary school was the most tangible and healthy act I could do for myself. I've been extremely fortunate to grow up among food goddesses— my maternal grandmother, aunt, and mother are (all great cooks). I learned how to savor food and make others smile. It's my superpower and secret weapon. I've been experimenting with food since I was three years old. Flavor profiles and different cuisines were my favorite type of experiments, to my parents' displeasure, because their digestive systems were sensitive. It was the most fun science ever! There's nothing like it when you can cook and help others have a nostalgic experience. Nothing is more human than taking a bite of food and closing your eyes in pleasure because it feeds your stomach and soul. I regress. There was a time when I was so broken that I let everything that gave me joy die. It's ironic, considering my name is Joy. Cooking and my faith in God were those sacred things I couldn't bear to part with, mainly because they were such an integral part of me. I worried that if those disappeared, I, too, would disappear forever. I felt protective over them, something I could have for myself. The outpouring of cooking connected me in a way nothing else did, and it brought love to people and myself.

The act of cooking changed the course of my life forever. Cooking is constant when everything else is shifting. Cooking was my first love. It's breath and life, literally and figuratively. It was my first step toward healing my need to please. Now, as a therapist, I realize all the benefits of culinary therapy, grounding in our five senses and feeding ourselves and others, which are powerful and transformational. There's restorative power in connection with your body, mind, and spirit.

Fast-forward 15 years. I facilitate healing through psychotherapy, but culinary therapy has an incredibly special place in my heart. Below is a dish I made myself when I wanted to ground in my five senses, get lost in the methodical chopping, and enjoy the action of cooking to nourish my soul.

THE TOOL

Culinary therapy is a therapeutic model that uses food as the medium along with your five senses (see, hear, taste, touch, and smell) to help ground yourself back in your body and connect to your mind. It's especially effective for those recovering from divorce, domestic violence, sexualized trauma, grief, sleep disturbances, and dissociative symptoms because it's all-consuming and forces one to be present. The difference from other grounding is that there is an order to things; creating a framework you can always count on using gastronomy and repetitive movements such as kneading bread, chopping, and stirring, which are highly therapeutic. To demonstrate this tool, I'll use my favorite Thai noodle bowl recipe to walk you through a series of techniques that helped me move trauma through my body and reframe the way I look at food and myself.

STEP ONE: MAKE A GROCERY LIST.

Focus on this one dish to make it simple rather than a whole grocery haul, which can be overwhelming and socially exhausting.

INGREDIENTS- MAKE 1 LARGE BOWL

4 ounces soba noodles, high protein spaghetti, or whole wheat spaghetti

⅛ cup of purple cabbage

½ cup white cabbage

Two carrots peeled and grated

½ red bell pepper, sliced into thin strips

One tablespoon of chopped green onions

Five ounces thinly diced chicken breast or tofu (leftovers from the night before). Please make sure your tofu is drained of liquid, and then lightly sauté it with salt/pepper

Peanut dressing

Two tablespoons of vegetable or chicken broth

½ cup peanut butter

Three tablespoons white wine vinegar or rice vinegar

Three tablespoons toasted sesame oil

Three tablespoons reduced-sodium tamari or other soy sauce

Two tablespoons of agave, honey or maple syrup

One tablespoon of finely grated fresh ginger

Two garlic cloves, minced

Juice of 1 lime

Garnish

Sprinkle of coarsely chopped peanuts

Handful of cilantro, coarsely torn

One lime, sliced into wedges

Optional: for added heat, add sriracha or chili-garlic sauce

STEP TWO: TAKE THREE CLEANSING 4-COUNT BREATHS.

Breathe in through your nose, counting to four slowly.

Hold for four.

Slowly exhale through the mouth for four seconds and repeat two more times.

STEP THREE: SET THE STAGE AND GET MIS EN PLACE.

Mise en place is a French culinary phrase that means "putting in place." It means preparing your space and yourself for the act of cooking. It's timesaving and helps order your mind. Get all your ingredients and equipment out before you start.

STEP FOUR: ACTIVATE THE SENSES.

As you prepare, chop, cook, serve, and taste this dish, experience it through your senses. You hear the crunch of the chef's knife through the cabbage as you dice or the crispness of the carrot against the grater. You smell the umami of the peanut sauce as it blends. You feel the cool texture of the red bell pepper as you core and slice. You see this colorful dish before you. You taste that first awaited bite and savor it.

STEP FIVE: COOK.

Set a large pot on the stove with water an inch from the top and set it on high to boil for noodles. Meanwhile, chop and slice the vegetables on a large cutting board with a chef's knife. I like to fine dice cabbage, grate carrot, thinly slice red bell, and chop green onions to include the green part. Check your water, place your noodles in, set an eight-minute timer, and take the lid off. I use a tiny ninja or food processor for the peanut sauce, but you can use a bowl and whisk just the same. Place ingredients for the sauce in and pulse three times (or whisk) till smooth. Slice limes, cut protein, and chop peanuts for garnish.

STEP SIX: ASSEMBLE AND TASTE.

Place the cooked noodles, protein, sauce, and vegetables in a serving bowl, toss until combined, garnish, and enjoy. Yum!

STEP SEVEN: BE GRATEFUL.

Gratitude can change your negative mood or mindset. Be intentional and grateful that you have taken a step to nourish your soul and prove trust and compassion to yourself by grounding in this moment. I say a simple prayer to God, "Thank you for providing this meal, restoring me, and loving me, amen."

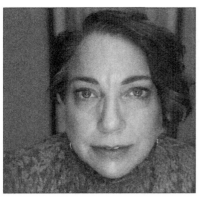

Joy E. Davis, LMSW, is the owner and therapist for JoyFULL Therapy, where she helps you heal your heart, mind, and spirit. You'll feel empowered to step out of your pit into your purpose. Her therapeutic focus is trauma recovery for individuals, families and couples. Joy thrives in helping others overcome conflict and communication barriers within their relationships and healing from divorce and religious hurt. Joy is also a pastoral consultant providing therapeutic guidance to pastors and church leadership for specialized support to prevent compassion fatigue while also guiding them in handling challenging situations through a trauma informed lens which is preventive to church hurt.

Joy is an entrepreneur, coach, and enthusiastic culinary therapist with two decades of immersive experience in the food industry. As a seasoned nutrition coach and health & wellness advocate, she blends the artistry of culinary skill with psychology to nourish the mind, body, spirit, and emotional well-being.

Joy has a culinary certificate from the renowned Culinary Institute of America, a Bachelor's degree in Psychology, and a Master's degree in Social Work. Joy has helped thousands of individuals heal and eat well. Joy had the honor of unique culinary experiences, including cooking for and organizing a Wounded Warrior event with former President George W. Bush.

Join me on the restorative healing and wholeness journey for more tips or therapeutic support. Check out the JoyFULL Therapy Website: https://joyedavis.com and JoyFULL Transformation Institute for memberships, courses, and more at https://linktr.ee/joyfulltherapy. Connect with me at https://www.psychologytoday.com/profile/1234575 for a free 20-minute consultation. Always on the move, Joy is creating therapeutic wellness retreats using culinary therapy and somatic movement to help participants deepen their joy, coming in 2025.

CHAPTER 15

INSTRUMENT OF PEACE

HOW CAN ONE REIKI SESSION CHANGE YOUR LIFE?

Carolyn Nicholson Fowler, URMT, KRMT®, NREMT-P, CRCC, CMRM

MY STORY

The first time I ever heard about Reiki, three of us stood around my son's hospital bed in January 2009: his wife Joy, her friend Renee (the Reiki master), and me. Renee asked us to close our eyes and visualize blue-green flames around him on the bed. Those were the healing colors. And because I'm a rebel, never doing as told, I peeked at the bed, and for the first time in my life, I saw the energy flowing in those colors around him! Over the next few days, I felt him both in and out of his body and knew he was conversing with God about whether to stay or leave. Five days later, my son died. The son who was like me and who had the same irreverent sense of humor, my Jon-Jon. I was shattered. All the colors and flavors left my life. I felt like a cardboard cutout. The days were gray. My other two children kept me grounded and semi-sane. Without them, I doubt I would've survived.

After his death, the world cruelly carried on. I got a not-exactly generous two days of bereavement leave, and I was walking around with a grief so deep, so profound, it felt as if there was a giant, bloody hole in my chest where my heart was supposed to be. I had no idea how, or even if, I could heal from it. This continued for a few months until I finally heard my angels and guides, who were likely screaming at the top of their lungs, *Try Reiki!* I remembered Renee, the Reiki Master, and called her to do some Reiki with me. I had no idea what to expect. I never heard of Reiki before that day in my son's hospital room, but I was searching anywhere for help with all the pain.

She set up her table and had me lie down. She took a few minutes to get ready. She was praying for our protection and setting the intention for the session. As soon as she laid her hands on my head, grief **roared** out of me like a jet engine. I felt it flying out of my hands and feet, and I sobbed uncontrollably. After a minute or so, that calmed a bit, and she moved her hands to a different position, and it started all over again. Intense doesn't come close to describing this session. I had no idea how long she worked with me—I wasn't even on this planet. Eventually, she brought me back to the present, and as I sat up on the table, I realized I could finally breathe! I hadn't been aware of being unable to breathe, but suddenly, I could take a deep breath, which felt amazing. It was as if an iron band around my chest had broken! I was awed by Reiki's power and the calmness I felt after one session. I decided then and there that I'd learn all I could about this powerful healing modality!

As I continued reading everything about Reiki I could get my hands on, it became evident I was being guided by an intelligence far surpassing mine. There was an almost instantaneous gut reaction to ego-based books, which said theirs was the only true Reiki, or you had to "Do it this way, or it won't work," all of which is untrue. Reiki is Reiki. It's an energy from the highest realm. It nourishes your entire life, starting with your soul. You're acting as a conduit. You plug in, and it comes through you. It's focused by your hands and intention, like prayer on steroids! The most important thing we do is to try to get out of our own way. We must take the ego out of our practice and try not to overthink it.

At this point, I'm sure you're wondering what Reiki is. I've been practicing and teaching it for 15 years, and that's very difficult to answer because it's different for everyone. In all the time I've practiced with hundreds of clients, I've only had two people react as profoundly and intensely as I did. I can only surmise that was because they were totally ready to release what needed to go. Every person who comes for a Reiki session has a different set of needs—a complex makeup of spiritual, mental, emotional, and physical issues. Reiki works with them all (on all levels). Because of my first experience with Reiki, I specialize in grief work, but despite the practitioner's intent, Reiki is intuitive, going where the need is greatest, and can never do harm. Some commonalities of how people feel after receiving a Reiki session are a profound sense of peace, feeling more relaxed and lighter, more restorative sleep, pain relief, greater clarity of thought, better balanced, and the ability to cope with life better. Practitioners train to feel the energy densities, indicating where energy is stagnated or stuck. We get the energy moving again, so the flow is back to being optimal for health. I love that we don't even have to touch the client! This can all be accomplished by moving the energy in their aura. Practitioners find they are less angry, more patient, more forgiving, and much calmer after practicing Reiki.

The results of research done with medical Reiki are startling. It's documented that there is less blood loss during surgery, less post-surgical pain, more stable blood pressure during surgery, and accelerated healing. This Reiki I practice (and teach) was brought to us by a Japanese man, Mikao Usui, born in 1865. He studied many things and traveled extensively, but in 1922, at age 57, he felt he had not found his true purpose. Frustrated, he decided to go up to the top of Mount Kurama, a holy mountain in Kyoto Prefecture, and meditate until he found answers. He spent over 20 days there, fasting and meditating, and over those days, received many epiphanies (we call them downloads; information from our guides and the Creator.) When he came down from the mountain, he was excited to share the visions and revelations he was given. He opened a school (dojo) and started teaching Reiki as a spiritual practice that healing was a part of. In 1923, there was a catastrophic earthquake in Tokyo. He and his students entered the city and started healing people on the spot. As you can imagine, interest in Reiki as a healing modality burgeoned, and as a result, Usui Sensei opened a larger clinic in Nakano. Usui passed away in 1926, and since then, many schools of Reiki have sprung up, each with its own essence, but all great healing tools and an endlessly fascinating and deep subject to study.

A quick story about how powerful this energy healing modality is: A former student knew a young man in the southeastern US who contracted a fungal infection in his lungs. He was in a prestigious hospital, and they worked for months to rid him of the fungus in his lungs, to no avail. At this point, he was on a ventilator and an ECMO (extracorporeal membrane oxygenation machine) to help oxygenate his blood. When my former student called me, the hospital was talking about palliative care for this man. I immediately thought that was the same as hospice, but the young man corrected me by saying it was to allow a different medical team into his care. At this point, his kidneys were also failing. I called on ten of my students who are Reiki Master Teachers (RMT), and we began a concerted effort to strengthen him and heal his lungs. This occurred in July 2023. In August, one month after the tsunami of Reiki energy was sent to him, his body encapsulated the fungal infection. He tested negative for the infection, which had to happen for him to be placed on the transplant list! We continued sending Reiki, and he slowly started getting better. In September 2023, he received a double lung and kidney transplant! He was weaned off the ECMO machine and the ventilator. He beat septic shock, aspergillus fungal infection, kidney failure, lung failure, and many other issues! This incredible young man was able to go home before Thanksgiving after 146 days (about five months) in the ICU!

Reiki, in addition to healing you as it passes through you, will hone your innate intuitive abilities. Many unique and unusual events happened after I committed to learning and doing Reiki. About two years after my son's death, I was walking through my living room with a cup of coffee in my hand. It was a gorgeous sunny morning outside with birds singing. My heart was so peaceful when something made me stop in my tracks. I literally stopped walking and asked myself: *What is going on with me?* I felt so different! *What on Earth? Oh my God, I'm happy!* It had been a long time since I felt happiness! That was a landmark day. A few months after that, walking again through my living room, I smelled my son's cologne. I now know that it was evidence of a visit from him!

THE TOOL

Now, to the tool I'm leaving you with to nourish your soul and life! You may have experienced over the last few years as if chaos and violence are everywhere. I teach my students a great way to shield themselves energetically against the harsh energies in the world. We do this every day, in the morning before starting our day. This is a two-part strategy.

First, we brush off the energies we have picked up in the world that we don't want to cling to us. Starting at your left shoulder with your right hand, you sweep your hand down and across your body to your right hip and fling that energy off! Next, the same movement starts on your right shoulder with your left hand. The shoulders carry all our 'shoulds'; who wouldn't like to eliminate a few of those? Then, holding your left arm out rigidly, sweep down the top of that arm with a flat hand, flinging off that energetic debris, then down the side of the arm in the same manner. Next, do the same with the right arm. Then lean over and brush off your legs down to your feet. This technique is known as Kenyoku Ho. Kenyoku is dry bathing in Japanese, and Ho means 'method', so you clean off before sealing yourself up to deflect all negative energy.

Next, we learn the shielding part. We begin by drawing a large Cho Ku Rei (pronounced cho koo ray) Reiki symbol with our entire hand in the air over the floor in front of us. Cho Ku Rei is the power and focus symbol, which is healing, protective, and powerful. We start by drawing a large number seven. From the bottom of that seven, we draw out, and to the right, a large circle that crosses the stem of the seven about three-quarters of the way to the top, becoming a spiral, getting progressively smaller, with three circular spirals over the central stem of the seven. With the smallest circle, the last of it will barely cross the upright part of the seven. If you are a visual learner, just google Cho Ku Rei, and study its form. Now you have created the Cho Ku Rei energy on the floor right before you! Step into it, bend over, pull that delicious energy up around you, and seal it over your head with gassho or prayerful hands. The intention you might use for this is, "No negativity will find me today, or no harm or negative thoughts will come to me today." You're shielded from harsh energies for the day now!

This is how one session of Reiki can change your life, as it did mine. It helped me heal from profound grief and brought me to a life of joy and purpose. Most of my clients become students. All of my students become friends. Reiki helps make you a better person with higher levels of self-pride and integrity. You notice others more and are more willing to give them grace when needed. Reiki will show you the way to a beautiful life.

I hope this has helped you, and that if you have any questions, you'll reach out to me!

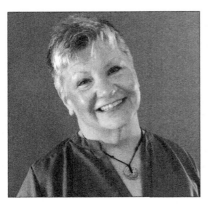

Carolyn Nicholson Fowler is a Usui Reiki Master Teacher and a Karuna Reiki® Master Teacher, Certified Medical Reiki Master, founder of the Peaceful Healing School and owner of Peaceful Healing Reiki LLC. She teaches all levels of intuitive Reiki, from Level One to Master Teacher. A former paramedic and doctor office MA, she brings a wealth of medical knowledge to her practice of Reiki. Carolyn is a medical intuitive, and channels angelic messages for clients. She partners with a local no-kill animal shelter, Satchel's Last Resort in Sarasota, Florida, to teach animal reiki. She is available for speaking engagements for groups about energy healing and griefwork.

A good friend of the late Raven Keyes, who authored *The Healing Power of Reiki* and *Medical Reiki, A Groundbreaking Approach to Using Energy Medicine for Challenging Treatments*, Carolyn became a certified Medical Reiki Master through Raven Keyes Medical Reiki International and is mentioned in the *Medical Reiki* book.

Reiki is the gentle, powerful, intuitive energy modality that balances and relaxes the body so it can heal itself. It helps with sleep, anxiety, grief, pain relief, PTSD, and too many more to mention. She practices hands-on and hands-off Reiki, described as "Relaxation for the Soul." Carolyn brings the study of Reiki to you with passion, humor, and fun!

You can reach her through her website:
https://peacefulhealingreiki.com

Instagram - https://www.instagram.com/carolyn17325

Facebook - https://www.facebook.com/carolyn17325

Email - carolyn17325@gmail.com

CHAPTER 16

WHEN RAINE CAME

SYNCHRONICITY, SURRENDER, AND THE TESTS OF INITIATION

Rev. Susan Wallace Donegan, RN

MY STORY

The twins were born exactly three months early. An ambulance ride in a snowstorm and five days of IV medication did nothing to slow down the arrival of these Aquarian ladies. The level-3 ultrasounds confirmed that there was no longer blood flow going to twin one, and an emergency C-section was performed. Rhiannon came weighing one pound 14 ounces. Raine came next at two pounds two ounces. I was present as the cardiologist was checking Rhiannon's heart with an ultrasound, commenting on what I knew as a registered nurse as I watched. I asked if the doctor had seen Raine yet, and by his abrupt reaction, I knew something wasn't good. "I have to speak to the parents first," he said.

"My daughter is exhausted. She can't hear bad news right now," I reminded the doctor. He began drawing me pictures of Raine's heart. The twins were mirror-imaged, meaning all of Raine's organs were on the opposite side of Rhiannon's. In addition, her heart had not formed correctly, with little in the way to be able to function outside her mother's womb. At most, he predicted, Raine wouldn't survive more than 48 hours. She was now on a ventilator in a quiet NICU, waiting for the inevitable. I was stunned. I had gone into nursing with a specialty in Labor and Delivery, and I could see how impossible this situation was, yet something in me needed to fight. And I hoped Raine would fight with me.

I was trained in several healing modalities: I was a Reiki master teacher, and recently trained in another healing modality called attunement, which accesses the endocrine system rather than the chakra system. I recently returned to work as a public health nurse following a leave of absence to work for Harvard Medical School's Department of Health Care Policy. I traveled the country testing an assessment tool for admission to rehab hospitals, which, for the first time, included medical conditions as well as physical ailments. This clarified the way those hospitals were reimbursed. The leave was granted, as it was quite an honor to be invited to this study for my rural New York State County. Now I'd have to ask for a leave again, as I was going to stay at the hospital. I found it interesting that I'd wandered into Sunrise Ranch on a whim, where attunement was taught (and is now a part of my skill set). It became my main tool when working with Raine.

I also called Harvard back to ask whether there was another possible outcome for Raine. Dr. Richard Jonas called back. "There's a surgery we can do called an arterial switch with reconstruction." Unfortunately, her heart was too small to be successfully worked on, and she was not a candidate for transplant, needing the same opposite alignment. If we could grow her to five pounds, he could do the surgery. That became the plan.

Rhiannon appeared to be healthy, and she was placed in a Feeders and Growers NICU. Raine, on the other hand, was in the Critical Care NICU. IVs and the ventilator, monitors, and bells were part of her daily life as I put my hands to work. The familiar energy moved through me and out to her, and she made it past the first 48 hours. The twins were fed through nasogastric tubes with a protein-rich formula with extra calories and breast milk. But preemie bowels often cannot handle that load, and Raine soon came down with NEC (Necrotizing Enterocolitis), where the bowel inflames, and feeding must be stopped. Treatment was usually surgery, but Raine was too fragile to tolerate that. Babies all around her were dying of the same. I took off the malachite heart necklace I wore and placed it in her incubator. Malachite is a great heart stone.

Raine was to experience NEC three more times with feeding being stopped. She was too fragile to be held, even by her mother. Her oxygenation fell with any movement, and often, her ventilator settings had to be increased in order to get her back. At those times, I was asked to leave the NICU as the code progressed. But I knew it was important I stay and hold the energy, so I identified my clergy status and was allowed to stay. I practiced visualizing rocking her in my arms and singing Sweet Baby James, injecting her name as I silently sang.

On a glorious day when the twins were eight weeks old, I happened to be present when the nurse asked if I wanted to hold Raine as she changed the incubator. "Absolutely!" Out came this little feather of a baby, lines, tubes, and all, and I took the opportunity to sing that song out loud as I rocked her. Her oxygen saturation climbed up and up until it was at 100%, and I was able to hold her for over an hour! How this tiny infant—too weak to open her eyes—heard my silent singing was a lesson I wouldn't forget. I was getting proof that there was more at work than even I knew.

Rhiannon grew steadily, and the time came for her to go home. As I made plans to buy her a nice outfit to go home in, we were called into the doctor's office. "Raine has come down with bacterial meningitis and probably won't make it through the night." We were devastated. I left my daughter and her partner to stay with Raine and went to the store for the outfit. I couldn't take in that this baby, who became precious to me, wasn't going to survive. I was exhausted from my efforts at constant energy healing and now grief, and I collapsed on the floor of that fancy store, wailing out my hurt to the salesgirl who rushed over. "Do I buy T-shirts for Raine or a christening gown to bury her in? A single stroller or a double?" The salesgirl took me to Rhiannon's nice outfit, then T-shirts and a double stroller, stating, "Now you get back to that hospital. That baby needs you!"

By the time I got back, Raine's tiny body had turned black. She was in a state of DIC (Disseminated Interstitial Coagulation), the body's last-ditch effort to save itself. And I was hit with the realization that all of my efforts at healing her were selfish. I felt my heart break as if it were glass, and I started praying. Hard. "God, please take her peacefully and Love her. I'm so sorry for holding onto her for so long." And the glass pieces of my heart fell to the floor.

And then I stood in a column of white light in the middle of that NICU. A power that was not my own began pouring into the crown of my head and out my arms, and my hands went to work pulling heat off of that baby. It went on for about an hour before I was exhausted. I lay down in the room next to her and was awakened about every two hours to return and work again. In the morning, Raine had no more signs of meningitis. She had been healed by that heavenly intervention. And never again did I take credit for any healing that happened through my efforts. So, I was healed as well.

But trouble was not over. The DIC left her hand with no circulation, and the ends of her fingers died. She was still too fragile to be taken to the OR for removal. The decision was made to allow them to just fall off. And, because she couldn't complain about pain, the National Infant Pain Scale came into play, where babies who couldn't rate their pain were medicated. Raine was put on morphine, and I could no longer reach her energetically with the healing modalities I used. She was drugged beyond my reach. Any effort to address with the doctors who, while they admitted my work had certainly made a difference in Raine's survival, that Infant Pain Scale was what they were following, and the morphine continued. Raine started to decline.

A decision was made that it was now or never for Raine's heart surgery. Enter again Dr. Richard Jonas, one of only three surgeons in the world who could perform Raine's surgery. He decided to take her at her four-and-a-half pounds rather than wait any longer, and she was flown by helicopter up to Boston Children's Hospital. Her surgery was a success! Yet still, the issue of pain from surgery and the fingers falling off kept her on morphine. Though I had some verity through my work for Harvard, the Infant Pain Scale still was in play, and I couldn't make that stop. Dr. Jonas felt that he might have to take Raine back to the OR, as her heart could not regain its normal rhythm. And then Heaven stepped in again.

On a day I wasn't present, a nurse was called away to a cardiac code as she was drawing up Raine's morphine. When she returned, she forgot to dilute the medication and gave her a lethal dose. As Raine coded, the nurse realized what happened and told the doctor, allowing for a reversal of the overdose. But Raine was back on the ventilator and declining. This nurse met me as I stormed in, explaining through tears what had happened and how horrible she felt. I saw her then as the nurse who sang to Raine and called me when I wasn't there to sing to her at night, and I forgave her and said, "Now take me to your supervisor."

With that came a meeting of the doctors and staff. I explained that I could no longer reach Raine with the morphine, and she was declining. They countered with the fact that I couldn't fix her heart using attunement, Reiki, and prayer. "Yes," I said. "But I got her here." And then, with the courage building in me through all of the apparent synchronicities, the healing in the NICU, and the promptings of Spirit, I found myself saying, "It goes my way, or I see a lawyer. You killed that baby."

We agreed upon a plan where I would use attunement, and know within five minutes whether I could alleviate the pain. If I couldn't, I'd allow a small amount of morphine to be given. They agreed. Raine received one tiny dose of morphine the next day and then no more. Her heart regained its rhythm, no more trips to the OR, and she was well on her way to healing and growing.

As Raine was preparing to be discharged from the hospital, Dr. Jonas came out and said, "I've been watching you, and I want to know what you've been doing." We had a long talk about the complimentary medicines, and he instituted a Reiki program for any nurses who wanted to learn. I also was informed that he changed, through Harvard's Department of Health Care Policy, the Infant Pain Scale. And Reiki is a certified nursing intervention. Not bad for a micropreemie to change the world, eh?

Rhiannon and Raine are now 23 years old. Both have attended college. Though Raine has mild MS, you could never tell as her unbridled joy is apparent to all who know her. And in retrospect, I have come to recognize the many synchronicities that allowed me to participate as I did in these arenas I never saw coming. From the chance job with Harvard, the meeting of the emissaries who teach attunement, and the mistakes made by the medical institutions that allowed for change to be made for the growth of all involved, I am grateful. And gratitude, that morning prayer of "Put me where you want me and guide my hands always," is the beginning of high vibrational work each day.

Two stories I'll tell about my magnificent Raine, who was so aware despite her fragility that it astounds me. As a toddler riding in the car with me one day, Sweet Baby James came on the radio. Raine exclaimed, "That's my song!" *Yes, Love, it is.* As a toddler again, she came skipping by me one day as I was visiting. She stopped short in front of me and climbed on my lap. She began pulling out that malachite heart that had long before been returned to me and was now hidden on its chain beneath my shirt. She studied it intensely, then looked at me. Back and forth a few times between the heart and myself before kissing it, then me, and hopping away. It still raises the hair on my arms. There is more to see than meets the eye, and as I maintain the practices of gratitude, prayer, joy, kindness, and all the things that raise our vibrational rate, I see so much more.

THE TOOL

Our ability to see beyond what is obvious to the eye is contingent on what our vibrational rate is. In raising and maintaining a high vibrational rate, I teach the things that have worked for me. Here at Wellspring, we look at and teach the maintenance of high vibrational living as being key to being able to proceed and look beyond what is presented, with the knowledge, as in Raine's story, of all things being ordered and fostered by the Universe, who truly does wish us all to succeed.

Try these and see what works for you:

Set a daily intention. Make it one in which you ask to put your best foot forward. If there is a personal intention that is present, ask for the highest and best goals for *everyone* involved.

Service work always raises your vibration. Be available, when appropriate, to offer a hand, a prayer, or a smile. Change your thoughts when they sway to anger or meanness. They do not serve your highest purposes. When faced with troubling situations or persons, examine whether they are placed perhaps to help your growth rather than hinder you. It's often the case that those troubling times are our biggest teachers when seen in that light.

Trust that the Universe is on your side, not only in your wishes and dreams but in the highest good for all. When we become aligned with this, life truly holds fullness in whatever we do, and our vibration is raised to levels where confusion no longer takes hold.

Pay attention to diet and restriction of substances that lower vibration, as well as what you feed your minds and bodies through communication and thought.

The tests of initiation into this higher realm where healing and an increased vision are accessed become part of you. Ask and you shall receive. All is well on the other side with the recognition that all is possible when you are working with, rather than against, the Universe.

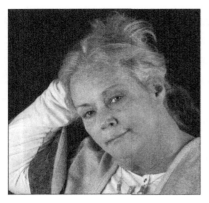

Rev. Susan Wallace Donegan is a Reiki Master Teacher, a trained practitioner in Attunement, and a Healing Touch, Remote Viewing, and shamanic practitioner trained in New York, Ireland, and Ecuador. She teaches out of her Wellspring office in Norwich, New York. She's a mother of five, grandmother of ten, and great-grandmother of four. She has been an intern for the Northern Cheyenne Grandmother of the 13 Indigenous Grandmothers. An interfaith minister in the Order of Melchisedek and The Center for the Living Earth, she is adopted as a Northern Cheyenne sister and grandmother. She has been in Montana lately, working to locate victims of the Missing and Murdered Indigenous People. It's her honor to be able to represent the Wittenburg Center at the United Nations for the Permanent Forum on Indigenous Issues and Women's Status.

Connect with Susan via email: wallacesue212@gmail.com.

CHAPTER 17

CONQUERING NEGATIVE THOUGHTS

NOURISH YOUR SOUL WITH MINDFULNESS MANTRAS

Daryl L. Mountford, RN, BSN

"What you habitually think largely determines what you will ultimately become."

~ Bruce Lee, Martial Arts Specialist/Actor

MY STORY

"You are what you think!" Let that sink in for a moment.

While "You are what you eat" is more common, both are equal and true. The thoughts we tell ourselves empower us and help us reach new heights, or they tear us down, leaving us full of self-doubt and anxiety. The universe brings us lessons to learn while here on this planet, and I was to come face to face with what mindful thinking was all about.

About 12 years ago, I began dealing with a serious medical diagnosis. I was suddenly facing an uncertain future and a lot of change. Not being one to shy away from difficulty, I believed I'd bravely handle anything thrown in my path. The reality of my journey was quite the opposite. I traveled down many steep and bumpy roads before understanding the true power of my internal dialogue. The outcome made me stronger and braver than I had ever been.

"From your lab results, it looks like we're dealing with rheumatoid arthritis," stated my rheumatologist in a flat voice. The nurse in me was five steps ahead of the conversation. The practical side of my brain was in high gear, deciding on an action plan.

Okay, you knew this was the most likely outcome. What meds will he put me on? How often will I need blood drawn? Will I need to adjust my schedule if the pain doesn't subside? How do I tell my mom without her worrying too much?

Having been a nurse for over ten years, I knew the damaging effects of RA and the medications for it on the body. I took care of many patients whose bodies were ravaged by the disease, so I was fully aware of where I could potentially be one day.

"What do you recommend for medications?" I asked directly, wanting facts and answers.

"Let's start with Plaquenil and Methotrexate and see how you feel in a month. Does that sound reasonable?"

While my physician was younger than me, he was quite reserved. Despite my best efforts, I couldn't get him to crack a smile. However, I liked that he respected my profession and wanted to tackle my prognosis as a team. He was proactive in his treatment and aimed to get ahead of the disease as quickly as possible. He answered all my questions thoroughly, and we formulated a plan.

"How do you feel?" he asked before we ended the appointment.

"Okay, relieved that I have an answer for all the pain and fatigue I've been feeling."

I answered honestly, but a large part of me didn't feel anything. I was still processing emotions. I'm hardwired with a glass-half-full outlook on life. I'll search for the silver lining in any challenging situation. Even with this diagnosis, I was determined not to pity myself or think, *why me?*

My mom and I have a running joke that if someone in the family is going to get sick with something unusual, it would be me. I overcame other illnesses and injuries in the past, so I did my best to look at this in the same light—one more thing to tackle and overcome.

I was 39 years old, single, working the night shift as a nursing supervisor, and dealing with nearly constant achy, stabbing pain in my hands and hips. I had days where simple tasks such as writing or typing had me in tears. My fingers were swollen, stiff, and sore, making holding a pen nearly impossible. The fatigue was bone-deep and more debilitating than the pain. It didn't matter how much rest or sleep I got; it was never enough. The pain either kept me awake or woke me up frequently, so sleep was never recuperative.

I stayed in bed until the last possible moment before I had to get ready for work. Many nights, it was a sheer struggle to get up. It was a tug-of-war with my body screaming to lie back down and my mind digging its heels in. My mind had a sense of duty to the patients and staff to be present regardless of what I was feeling. I managed to get to work most shifts from complete stubbornness.

About a month after starting the medication, I started to feel some relief from the amount of pain, and the joints in my fingers were less swollen. While this was positive, I struggled internally. I shared the news with my family and close friends, keeping it mainly to the facts and not confiding how I truly felt. On the outside, I had my shield up and appeared ready for battle, but I was falling apart on the inside.

Each passing day found negative emotions tiptoeing in, creating a circuit of doubt in my thoughts. I could barely get through a day without pain and wondered, *how am I going to handle a lifetime of this?*

What if my symptoms get worse? Will I be able to take care of myself? I'm all alone. How am I going to manage?

The nights I worked kept my mind occupied and didn't allow for pessimistic thoughts. But when I was off, my mind was riddled with anxiety, and uncertainty overflowed. I slept as much as possible to silence the messages. I was depressed and paralyzed, not knowing how to move forward. My thought pattern froze as a one-track path of doom and gloom. Somewhere along the way, I lost my ability to find a glimmer of good in my life.

Most days were a blur of physical pain and mental exhaustion. I was on automatic pilot, wanting to bury myself in routine because I didn't have the mental or emotional capacity to process anything outside of the norm. I cried more in the few months after my diagnosis than I had in my entire life. There is no cure for RA. It is a lifelong illness that is a continuous balancing act of all the aspects of your life.

Where do I even start?

I decided to join an online support group for people with RA. It was immensely comforting to know I wasn't alone in my suffering. I didn't contribute much, but I read many posts and articles people shared. I realized I was in a far better place physically than many of the members. As difficult as it was, I could still go to work and be productive. A lot of members felt guilty and defeated because they couldn't care for their families as they used to. I was lucky to have only myself to care for.

Around the same time, I read an eye-opening article about which foods could cause or exacerbate inflammation. There were specific foods mentioned to avoid if you had RA, some surprising to me. I knew how healthy food nourished the body from years of teaching patients about a cardiac diet, but I was enlightened about food nourishing you mentally and emotionally.

While having coffee with a close friend, I had an aha moment of clarity. I shared with her how many of the support group posts mirrored my thoughts.

"I know it must be extremely cathartic for people to express their emotions and let out their fears and anxieties, but there aren't many uplifting or empowering posts. I don't begrudge anyone for sharing them, but most are of the 'woe is me' variety."

"If they don't help you feel better, why do you go on then?" she asked, puzzled.

Her question stopped me in my tracks.

Wow! My brain is playing the same sob story soundtrack on repeat. Inside, I sound just like most of the posts. The needle is stuck in a groove, and I need to play another song!

It was an epiphany to realize I was feeding myself the same unhealthy thoughts as other people in the group. I was focused on what I *could* lose and not what I still had. My glass-half-empty attitude caused all the water to evaporate, and I needed to replenish my glass with positivity. The time for change was now. I wanted to sit in the light again, not in the shadows.

If food nourishes the body, thoughts are nourishment for the mind. I began analyzing my diet and what I fed my body. Rewiring how I talked to myself took a little more time. I began by concentrating on my accomplishments throughout the day and recognizing them as wins. I stopped focusing on the pain and what it stopped me from doing. The days when the pain was crippling were especially hard, but I knew if I kept a positive mindset, I'd feel better at the end of it.

Slowly, I shifted the narrative from *I can't* to *look what I did.* Thoughts become things, whether positive or negative. What we choose to focus on and tell ourselves becomes our reality. I was conscious of my internal dialogue; the more positive my thoughts were, the more positivity I attracted into my life. I learned to be more fully engaged and present in the moment.

I am so proud of you!

This simple but positive statement became my daily affirmation. I learned how practicing mindfulness kept me focused on the wins, big and small. Repeated messages of positivity reinforced my behavior and choices. Healthy decisions made me feel good, so I wanted to continue making them. Like choosing to eat healthy every day, it was vital for me to create a routine regarding what I told myself. Taking care of my thoughts while I was alone was key. A daily mindfulness mantra of positive thoughts enabled new pathways to form in my mind and sever the anxious, negative ones.

I choose to see the good in all situations.

I began to feel less stressed and anxious; a sense of inner peace and calm became the norm. I created a mindset of self-acceptance and compassion. Part of my mindfulness journey was allowing grace into my life and forgiving myself for past failures. I needed to let go of guilty feelings. I couldn't change the past, but could move forward with a new mindset. Change becomes more uncomfortable as we age. I learned to be kind to myself as I went through the process of shifting my internal messages. I didn't scold or blame myself if I slipped. I forgave and empowered myself for the next day.

I forgive myself for past failures and let go of the past.

I listen intently to my body when it whispers in my ear, telling me to rest. I don't ignore the screams anymore and embrace the well-deserved downtime. My mind and body now have a symbiotic relationship where they encourage each other and agree when we've done enough.

Over time, I reclaimed the armor of my inner warrior, forging it anew with each step forward. I felt stronger in every facet of my being than ever before. In addition to my shield, I carried a sword of positive energy to cut down the anxiety before it found a nook in my brain to nestle in and grow. I now look upon the future with a smile instead of tears.

I choose to face the challenging days with love and bravery. I control how I nourish my body temple physically, mentally, and emotionally. Living my life in the healthiest ways possible, in whatever capacity that looks like, is of the utmost importance. The vibrations of healthy eating and thinking have lifted my spirit. I feel lighter and more in tune with all areas of myself. Adopting mindfulness saved me, and it can help you, too. I planted positive seeds of encouraging thoughts, watered them daily, warmed them with self-love, and grew a lifetime's worth of positivity and strength. The best day for you to plant a garden is today.

THE TOOL

Choosing a mindfulness mantra that resonates with you, emphasizes what you wish to change, and evokes a sense of empowerment and self-awareness is essential. You want to feel the power and vibrations of the words as they uplift you. Set aside dedicated time to select your mantra and meditate on it. I find mornings are the best time for me as I can set the tone of my day.

Routine is crucial when first starting. Beginning a new healthy habit requires a lot of mental effort to stay the course. Stress and anxiety will try to interrupt these new habits and return to what's comfortable. Daily practice lets your mind automatically turn to light, encouraging thoughts rather than dark ones. You'll think, *Yes! I can do this!*

The beauty is you can do these throughout the day, multiple times if needed. If you're having a particularly trying day, carve out five minutes in a quiet place to reset your mind and thoughts. There is no one-size-fits-all with this tool. Use it in whichever way works for you.

Playing nature sounds while meditating with my mantra helps me relax and be in the moment. If you have music you enjoy, play it in the background to enhance your experience. Make the moment yours and own it.

PREPARATION:

1. Find a comfortable place where you can sit and relax. Be sure it's a place without distractions, and you can be fully present and engaged.

2. Take a deep breath in. Hold it for a count of four and release it slowly.

3. Decide which mantra you will use as you let your limbs relax.

   SAMPLE MANTRAS:
   a. I trust in my ability to handle any situation that arises.
   b. I am good enough, just as I am.
   c. I am proud of myself.
   d. I am present in this beautiful moment.
   e. I am worthy of love, peace, and happiness.

4. Take in another deep breath. Hold it for a count of four and release it slowly.

BEGIN:

5. Close your eyes and begin to say your mantra out loud or internally. Focus and be present with each word and what it means to you.

6. Continue to say your mantra for one minute. Be purposeful. You are feeding yourself nourishing thoughts.

7. Take deep breaths when necessary to keep yourself grounded and intent.

8. Evaluate how you feel after one minute. It's okay if you find your mind wandering. This is completely natural when we are stressed and anxious. Refocus, take another deep breath or two, and start again.

9. Repeat your mantra for another minute.

10. Once you feel ready, open your eyes, gently move your limbs, and come into the present moment. Now, go and tackle the day with positivity!

For more nourishing mindfulness mantras, please check out my website, www.messagesofmindfulness.com.

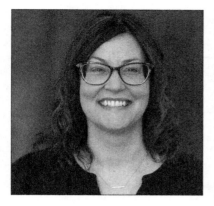

Daryl L. Mountford holds a Bachelor of Science degree in nursing from The Sage Colleges and a Bachelor of Science degree in biotechnology from Rochester Institute of Technology. She's also a certified tarot reader, certified crystal healer, and certified intuitive food therapist.

After 22 years of nursing in the cardiac field, Daryl retired in 2023 to begin a new chapter in her second love, writing and editing. She is the editor of Medium T. Brandon Russ's book, *Funny You Should Say That!* She owns 10th House Editing, a proofreading and editing company, and is the chief editor at 10th House Publishers. As chief editor, Daryl has shared her knowledge of writing through a class series, "Crafting Your Story."

A natural healer and empath, Daryl is inspired to help others heal on their journeys through life, utilizing her medical knowledge and intuitive gifts. When not reading or writing, she spends time with her family, friends, and two cat fur babies, Marble and Boo.

Connect with Daryl:

Facebook: https://www.facebook.com/DarylMountford

Instagram: https://www.instagram.com/10thhp

Email: Healingtarotwithdaryl@gmail.com

Website: https://www.10thhouseediting.com or www.10thhp.com

CHAPTER 18

NUMEROLOGY NUTRITION

THE SACRED PATH TO BALANCING YOUR BODY'S TEMPLE

Janet Namaste

MY STORY

From my earliest memories, sacred rituals were deeply steeped in my Russian immigrant family. Mealtimes were sacred rituals steeped in tradition, love, and vibrantly wholesome food. "You are what you eat" was one of the heartbeats of our traditions.

Although we lacked monetary wealth at that time, our real riches overflowed in the kaleidoscope of art, connection, and food prepared by caring, loving hands. My family invested generously in fresh ingredients; luxury was fresh flowers for the home. The greatest luxury for me was spending quality time together, time to share, time to savor every bite as sustenance for body, soul, and healing. I didn't know then how precious sharing those meals and family gatherings was, but I sure know it now.

Friday nights were my favorite when our small apartment was filled with 15-plus friends and relatives sharing a meal. I'd sit contentedly amid the belly laughs and the conversation's ebb and flow as multiple languages were spoken—Russian, Ukrainian, German, Romanian, Polish, Yiddish, and Hebrew. Though the words differed, the array of languages harmonized in a tapestry of love, resilience, and hope for future generations.

When dinner was over, I secretly waited for the invitation from the adults to play cards or dominos with them. I'd happily be swept into the elders' traditional card games, aware these were indeed lessons in numerology and energy readings disguised as fun. I was a curious student and quickly learned all the rules via visualization techniques, such as assigning colors to suit clubs/diamonds and tallying arithmetic values. Even at that young age, I instinctively knew there was a hidden order underlying all things and loved connecting the dots in all the techniques taught.

I was born with the gift of extrasensory abilities—clairvoyance, clairsentience, and clairaudience. From as early as I can remember, I perceived colors and energies radiating from each person's aura, instantly reading which chakras were open, blocked, or deficient. I read everyone's energy while playing cards and knew who was bluffing and who was telling the truth. Birthdays for me were no longer just dates but whole experiences etched in my consciousness by the vibrational imprint of each soul. Before we began playing, I always asked everyone's birthday, instinctively connected their numbers to color, and read their energy.

I experienced many personal healing journeys, but one that holds close to my heart was when I was 13 and watched my dad overworking and not honoring his body with good nutrition. When he turned 40, he was diagnosed with diabetes. He worked two jobs and slept only a few hours every night. During the day, he worked as a mechanical engineer for a large company. At 6 p.m., we'd share a family dinner, and shortly after, he'd begin his work for the company he was building. He desired to provide the best for his family while pursuing the American dream. But we rarely spent Friday night dinners with others, for he was building up a new business that took precedence and cost him his well-being.

Being able to see, hear, feel, and sense energy at 13 years old, I noticed that my dad's energy field was depleted. Having the "clair" discernment to read the energetic imprint of people's subtle energy fields, I sensed his aura was tethered. Through my psychic lens, it was obvious that certain chakras were gray, especially his second and fourth chakras.

My mother, an advocate of integrative medicine, began implementing a disciplined, nutritious, healthy diet for my dad. With her support, he began focusing once again on fitness, nutrition, and a healthy mindset.

My parents and many family members, including my children, are athletes. Discipline, working out, and meal prep are the norm in the household. He eventually sold his business and dedicated time to his healing journey. His diet included foods that fed his second and fourth chakras and his body as a whole. Was he cured of diabetes? No, but with the proper nutrition he embodied for his numerological soul essence and biological constitution, and with my mother's support, he chose healing and vitality. My signature program, The Destiny Blueprint, was born at that moment.

The Destiny Blueprint is a profound gift, and I'm deeply honored to guide countless individuals. I channel clients' pre-birth plans using universal laws, numerological insights, spiritual connection, and my clairvoyant abilities. Each session typically lasts four to five hours, revealing their gifts, challenges, Akashic records, and dharmic missions. Preparation consumes 20-30 hours per person, ensuring a tailored experience that respects their journey.

Through intense meditation, I tap into their soul essence, encompassing numerology, past lives, chakras, colors, and soul family, offering guidance for the next three years. Healing occurs authentically, as truth alone liberates. I intend to empower others by sharing this profound knowledge.

Inspired by my own and my family's healing journeys, I've dedicated myself to helping others unlock their inner wisdom for holistic well-being. My expertise in energy healing, nutrition, and numerology, coupled with life experiences, enables me to be an expert in translating cosmic insights. I've learned that every moment offers choices, shaping our mental, spiritual, and physical nourishment. Exploring my numerological essence empowers me to make informed decisions.

For me, numerology is the language of the divine. It's a way that Spirit connects with me and easily shows me the next step of my life's journey. The moment I embraced the relationship between numerology, colors, chakras, and nutrition, I began living in alignment with my life's highest destiny.

THE TOOL

Imagine being able to create a plate in a way that harmonizes with your soul essence number, fostering a deeper sense of inner peace and emotional equilibrium. Visualize yourself intuitively gravitating toward nourishing foods that align with your numerological essence, providing the perfect fuel to support and meet you wherever you are.

Everything vibrates in the cosmos with a unique energetic frequency, including numbers, colors, and chakras within our bodies. The interplay between numerology, color psychology, chakras, and nutrition weaves a rich, beautiful tapestry of holistic well-being. This ancient wisdom reveals a profound interconnectedness that you can use to nourish yourself on a deep, holistic level.

At the heart lies the quest for self-discovery and healing. You may find that the concepts of numerology and nutrition may seem completely unrelated, but when you consistently use this simple tool, you'll discover how they align. Numerology is an ancient system that assigns numerical values to words, names, and dates to uncover their influence and significance. On the other hand, nutrition is the biological study of the nutrients in food and how they nourish the body, our soul's temple.

This tool is simple as it marries the connection between your chakras, colors, soul essence, and numbers. It'll aid in nutritional tips to raise your energy vibration. Once you discover your key personal numerological blueprint behind your essence, life path, and lesson number you will be in awe of the brilliance that the universe provides. The affirmations and journal prompts are there to support your journey of spiritual numerological nutrition. Consistency with journaling and affirmation is key and will surely get you on the path of your highest potential.

THE UNION OF NUMEROLOGY AND CHAKRAS

Numerology is a system that assigns numerical values to words, names, and dates based on the teachings of the Greek mathematician Pythagoras. Pythagoras believed that the physical world was the amalgamation of the energetic vibrations of numbers and developed a system that corresponded letters with integers. Each single digit number from one to nine carries its vibrational essence and symbolic meaning.

The chakra system stems from Hindu traditions and represents the seven main energy centers aligned vertically along the spine. Each chakra governs specific emotional, physical, and spiritual elements of your being. When chakras become blocked or imbalanced, they can manifest as various issues, from low self-esteem to digestive problems.

According to the theories, numerology numbers directly correlate to specific colors and chakras:

1 - Red (Root Chakra)

2 - Orange (Sacral Chakra)

3 - Yellow (Solar Plexus Chakra)

4 - Green (Heart Chakra)

5 - Blue (Throat Chakra)

6 - Indigo (Third Eye Chakra)

7 - Violet (Crown Chakra)

8 - White (Higher Chakras)

9 - Gold (Higher Heart Chakra)

YOUR KEY NUMBERS FOR DISCOVERING YOUR NUTRITIONAL NUMEROLOGY

There are three primary numerological numbers to identify from your birthdate:

Essence Number - The day you were born.

Lessons Number - The month you were born.

Life Path Number - The sum of your birthday, month, and year.

Use this tool to calculate yours:

Birthday ____ (Essence Number)

Birth Month ____ (Lessons Number)

Birth Year ____ (Mission Number)

Essence Number = Birthday

Example: Born on the 21st, Essence Number = 21 = 2 + 1 = 3

Lessons Number = Birth Month Number

Example: Born in March, Lessons Number = 3

Life Path Number = Birthday + Birth Month + Birth Year

Then, reduce to a single digit.

Example: Born April 21st, 1988

Life Path = 4 + 21 + 1988 = 2013 = 2 + 0 + 1 + 3 = 6

Your Essence reveals your innermost nature and path to realign with your true self. Your Lessons highlight subconscious challenges to overcome. Your Life Path reflects your dharmic purpose and potential in this lifetime.

NUTRITIONAL GUIDANCE

Let's explore the beautiful correlation between numerology and its connections to color, chakras, and nutrition. As you unveil the essence numbers, month numbers, and their resonance with dietary choices, you will discover how you can begin harmonizing your body, mind, and spirit just by your awareness and putting gentle action into practice.

With this self-knowledge, you can use nutrition to reinforce the balanced vibrations of your personal numbers or provide counter-energies to areas needing development.

FIND YOUR NUTRITIONAL NUMEROLOGICAL BLUEPRINT:

Focus on your:

Soul Essence Number first - As your core self's nutritional foundation

Lessons Number Next - To unblock and integrate subconscious lessons.

Life Path Number - Supports fulfilling your dharmic calling and Higher Self's path.

STEP 1 - CALCULATE YOUR SOUL ESSENCE NUMBER

Your Soul Essence number represents your innermost nature and soul's purpose.

Your Soul Essence number is the day you were born. Your soul's essence is the expression of your innate being. This number reminds you of what the constitution is within your heart and soul and brings you back to yourself.

EX - Calculation of Essence: For example, if your birthday is January 16th, you would add 1 16 (day) = 1 +6 = 7. So, the essence number in this case would be 7.

STEP 2 - MONTH NUMBER

Your month number corresponds to the current phase and circumstances in your life. Use the number of the current month (January=1, February=2, etc.).

STEP 3 - UNDERSTAND THE NUMBER MEANINGS

Each single digit number carries specific vibrational qualities:

1 - Independence, Leadership

2 - Balance, Harmony

3 - Self-Expression, Creativity

4 - Stability, Persistence

5 - Adventure, Freedom

6 - Nurturing, Responsibility

7 - Spirituality, Analysis

8 - Abundance, Power

9 - Humanitarian, Completion

STEP 4 – ALIGN YOUR DIET

Look at the qualities of your essence and current month numbers.

- Choose foods that energetically resonate with those vibrations.
- For example, if your essence is 2 (harmony) and month is 6 (nurturing), eat grounding nourishing foods like leafy greens, nuts, whole grains.

STEP 5 – BE CONSISTENT + KIND TO YOURSELF

- Set aside time daily to journal about how you can embody the qualities of your numbers through your dietary choices.
- Use the affirmations stating your intention to align your nutrition with your numerological blueprint.

STEP 6 – NOTICE AND HONOR THE SUBTLE SHIFTS

- Remain open and aware of any changes in your energy, mindset, or well-being as you apply this practice consistently.
- Celebrate the sacred connection between numbers and your nutritional needs.

When you honor this simple practice of Numerology nutrition you awaken the vitality that is within your body, your soul, and spirit.

NUMBER MEANINGS AND NUTRITIONAL PRACTICES

1. THE GENESIS OF SELF (ROOT CHAKRA, RED)

Nourishing: Root veggies like potatoes, beets, proteins.

Unbalanced: Insecurity, disconnected from body.

Balanced: Grounded, stable, self-reliant.

Practice: Yoga, outdoor time, meditations for safety/security, root veggie dishes.

Journal: How can I feel more grounded and secure in my physical body today?

Affirmation: "I am a confident leader taking assertive action on my authentic path."

2. THE DANCE OF DUALITY (SACRAL CHAKRA, ORANGE)

Nourishing: Orange fruits/veggies like carrots, mangos.

Unbalanced: Creative blocks, emotional numbness.

Balanced: Passionate self-expression, intimacy.

Practice: Nurture creativity, relationships, sensual orange foods.

Journal: List out creative projects or hobbies that excite your passions.

Affirmation: "I embrace harmony by accepting all parts of myself and others."

3. THE SYMPHONY OF CREATION (SOLAR PLEXUS CHAKRA, YELLOW)

Nourishing: Whole grains, citrus fruits.

Unbalanced: Low self-esteem, digestive issues.

Balanced: Confidence, self-discipline.

Practice: Self-worth affirmations, creativity, sunny yellow foods.

Journal: About your favorite way of creative expression and why.

Affirmation: "I confidently communicate my truth and expansive ideas."

4. THE PILLARS OF STABILITY (HEART CHAKRA, GREEN)

Nourishing: Leafy greens, green veggies.

Unbalanced: Struggles with love, bitterness.

Balanced: Compassion, forgiveness.

Practice: Acts of kindness, gratitude, heart-nourishing greens.

Journal: Journal about an experience that opened your heart to giving/receiving more love.

Affirmation: "With an open heart, I cultivate stability, order, and renewal."

5. THE CATALYST OF CHANGE (THROAT CHAKRA, BLUE)

Nourishing: Hydrating teas, blue foods.

Unbalanced: Communication blocks, feeling unheard.

Balanced: Authentic self-expression.

Practice: Mindful communication, singing, throat-soothing liquids.

Journal: When was a time you spoke your voice with courage and clarity?

Affirmation: "I adapt with freedom, speaking my truth with clarity."

6. THE NURTURING HEART (THIRD EYE CHAKRA, INDIGO)

Nourishing: Nuts, seeds, plant proteins.

Unbalanced: Lack of intuition, headaches.

Balanced: Imagination, wisdom, insight.

Practice: Meditation, visualization, protein-rich mind foods.

Journal: Meditate on your intuitive wisdom and a vision for your spiritual journey.

Affirmation: "Through nurturing service, I cultivate wisdom and inner peace."

7. THE MYSTIC SEEKER (CROWN CHAKRA, VIOLET)

Nourishing: Pure, light foods.

Unbalanced: Disconnected from Spirit.

Balanced: Enlightenment, grace.

Practice: Meditation, prayer, fasting, purifying foods.

Journal: What are you grateful for that represents divine connection/consciousness for you?

Affirmation: "I surrender to the divine flow, experiencing enlightenment."

8. THE ABUNDANT HARVEST (HIGHER CHAKRAS, WHITE)

Nourishing: Whole grains, superfoods.

Unbalanced: Lack of purpose, scarcity mindset.

Balanced: Living your higher calling, prosperity.

Practice: Envisioning success, affirmations, wholesome abundance of foods.

Journal: Journal about your soul's calling and vision of abundant spiritual prosperity.

Affirmation: "I align with infinite abundance, manifesting success."

9. THE GATEWAY TO ENLIGHTENMENT (HIGHER HEART, GOLD)

Nourishing: Plant-based, high-vibration foods.

Unbalanced: Unforgiving, bitter.

Balanced: Unconditional love, compassion.

Practice: Selfless service, forgiveness, uplifting plant-foods.

Journal: List ways you can be of compassionate service today. What plant-based foods "love" all beings?

Affirmation: "With unconditional love, I serve others on my enlightened path."

Use these signs of chakra balance/imbalance as a guide. Then, implement the recommended nutritional practices and affirmations to harmonize your numbers' energies.

For example, if your Essence is 4 (heart chakra):

Regularly eat green leafy vegetables and vegetable dishes to nourish that chakra's energies of compassion and stability as your essence.

If your Lesson is 7 (crown chakra):

Notice if you feel disconnected spiritually and counter that by adding very light, pure foods like fasting or a simple vegetable-based diet to reawaken your enlightenment lessons.

If your Life Path is 9 (higher heart chakra):

Uphold your humanitarian life path by prioritizing a plant-based diet and a mindset of unconditional love to actualize that potential—Journal about the compassionate service you provide.

Be consistent with nourishing all three key numbers through nutritious, mindful practices. The more you embrace this holistic approach, the more profound insights will arise for your personal growth and radiant well-being.

The connection between numerology and nutrition offers a unique way to understand the profound impact of food and thought choices on your overall well-being. By aligning what you eat with the vibrational frequencies associated with your soul essence and month numbers, you can tailor your life to nurture harmony, balance, and vitality.

Rather than viewing food as mere sustenance, this ancient wisdom invites you to appreciate the energetic qualities imbued in every bite. Just as each number carries its distinct vibration, the foods and the thoughts you consume resonate with specific frequencies that can enhance or disrupt your energy field.

Throughout my life, I have experienced numerous personal healing journeys, including those close to my heart. My dad inspired this awakening in me with his healing journey, and since that day, I've incorporated numerological nutrition in all aspects of my life. The greatest gift I've been given is sharing this knowledge with you and the world. As I embrace my soul's essence as a number 4, I choose to love and share knowledge with compassion and generosity. I'm a true archetype of a teacher, student of the universe, and artist. It's a great joy to share this beautiful tool— a marriage of numbers, nutrition, chakras, colors, affirmations, journaling, and tips to honor the uniqueness of the love that you are. Embrace your soul's calling; embrace the tapestry of your beautiful journey. Shine bright, dear one!

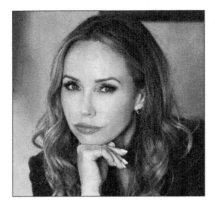

Janet Namaste is an intuitive healer and numerologist with over 25 years of professional experience who helps people discover their life's purpose, heal, and align to their destined path. Through her innate psychic and clairvoyant skills, she has guided thousands worldwide in discovering their life's purpose through her private sessions, programs, masterclasses, and workshops.

Janet has facilitated the healings of thousands globally utilizing her natural + nurturing skills as the four "clairs" (clairvoyant, claircognizant, clairaudient, clairsentient) and a Reiki Master. Through her private sessions, masterclasses, and group programs, she channels unique information for the transformation for the highest good of all. She's taught hundreds of workshops in the realm of energy healing, love, relationships, angels, numerology, family constellations, and more. She's also a skilled hypnotherapist specializing in regression therapy trained by world-renowned Dr. Brian Weiss, whom she met in 2000.

She is a spiritual teacher, thought leader, intuitive consultant, Host of *Raw Real Talks*, and founder of The Conscious Healer's Academy, an International program for healing professionals that helps raise the consciousness of the world and the Soul Star Membership, a nurturing community for all.

As an expert transformational coach, certified in Creativity in Business Master's Degree Program from Stanford University, Janet leads the NYC Stanford University Mindfulness Program, where she teaches privately and in the New York Board of Education.

In her numerous speaking engagements, Janet is known for her nurturing yet keeping it real candor. Her humorous and grounded delivery continues to inspire people globally. Whether through seminars or private consultations, Janet is highly praised for their natural ability to help people understand their life's purpose and develop practical strategies to remove blocks and align with the path of destiny and purpose.

Visit:

www.janetnamaste.com

Janet Namaste the Podcast – listen on all platforms

Social (IG, FB, YouTube) @janet.namaste

CHAPTER 19

SOUL SUSTENANCE

HIGH VIBRATIONAL EATING
FOR FREE FLOWING HEALTH

Chef Lisa Brown

MY STORY

In the shadow of a tumultuous upbringing, I found myself ensnared in a web of violence, addiction, neglect, and emotional abuse. Raised in a home where fear was a constant companion and love felt like a distant dream, I sought refuge in the only sanctuary I knew—food. As the chaos of my parents' battles echoed through the walls, I turned to food as a shield, using its comforting embrace to numb the ache in my soul. But with each bite, I found myself sinking deeper into the abyss, the numbness of my senses a poor substitute for the love and security that eluded me. With no healthy role models for love and no guiding lights to show me what a nurturing relationship looked like, I internalized the pain. Unbeknownst to me at the time, my connection with food was destined to transcend mere sustenance and would eventually evolve into a deep journey of self-discovery, healing, and, ultimately, free-flowing health.

My childhood was a tapestry woven with threads of pain and despair, each day a struggle to navigate the treacherous waters of my family's dysfunction. "I hate you! I hate you!" My mother's drunken slurs cut through the air like a knife, each word dripping with venom as she launched into a tirade against my father. A tormented soul haunted by his ghosts, my father lashed out with fists of fury, leaving behind a trail of broken hearts and shattered dreams. The stench of alcohol hung heavy in the air, mingling with the acrid scent of fear that permeated our home on a daily basis. My father's murderous outbursts toward my mother left my twin brother and me to carry the heavy burden of her pain as she unwittingly transferred her suffering onto us, although I endured the brunt of it. "I can't take this anymore," I whispered to myself, the words barely audible over the roar of my father's rage. *Why won't they stop?* I thought repeatedly. Each scream, each crash, felt like a dagger piercing my fragile heart, leaving behind wounds that would scar for life. Tears welled up in my eyes as I huddled in my room, seeking refuge from the storm that raged outside. *Please make it stop*. I pleaded silently, my voice choking with desperation.

In the eerie silence that followed the storm of violence, the air hung heavy with the weight of unspoken horrors. As I stood there, trembling in the aftermath, the scent of fear was palpable. My mind raced with memories of the brutality that just unfolded before me. I witnessed my father's relentless rage as he struck my mother with unyielding force, the sight etched into my memory.

"This can't be real," I muttered, my voice barely above a whisper, as if trying to convince myself that what I witnessed wasn't happening. I could still hear the sickening sound of her screams echoing through the halls, the sound of her body being dragged across the floor, leaving a trail of anguish in her wake. And then there were the objects—weapons of destruction wielded with reckless abandon in the heat of the moment. I remember the snow globe, thrown with such force it shattered upon impact, sending glass fragments flying through the air with a vengeance. The shards cut the back of my heel, leaving a lasting scar I carry to this day. *I can't deal with this right now*, I thought, my heart pounding in my chest, seeking some semblance of control amidst the chaos. In a desperate attempt to numb the pain, I reached for the nearest source of comfort I could find—the loaf of bread sitting on the kitchen counter.

Without hesitation, I tore into it, devouring slice after slice with reckless abandon, the taste of dough becoming a bittersweet distraction from the turmoil raging within me. But with each bite, the knot in my stomach tightened, the guilt and shame of my actions threatening to overwhelm me. I felt the familiar sensation of nausea creeping in, a physical manifestation of the emotional pain I tried so hard to suppress. As I doubled over in pain, the agony in my stomach served as a harsh reminder of the toll my actions took on both my body and soul. I couldn't help but wonder how I allowed myself to sink so low. Even in the midst of my despair, the hunger for relief (both physical and emotional) was insatiable, driving me to consume more and more until my stomach churned with sickness.

"This will make it all go away," I mumbled between mouthfuls, the taste of bread becoming a temporary distraction from the pain and confusion. The bread offered a fleeting escape, a momentary reprieve from my harsh reality. "I'm worthless," I told myself, a mantra of self-hate that echoed in the darkest corners of my mind.

Amidst the endless chaos and dysfunction that gripped our home, my mother's battle with bipolar disorder added another layer of complexity to our already tumultuous lives. Even after my father left for good, she continued to self-medicate, drowning her sorrows in alcohol and pills. I remember the days when she slept for what felt like an eternity, only to awaken in a rage that seemed to consume her entire being. The unpredictability of her moods was terrifying, like walking on eggshells around a ticking time bomb. She exploded into a fit of anger over the smallest of perceived slights. It was a constant rollercoaster of emotions, leaving us never knowing how she'd respond to our innocent childhood antics. Then there were the accusations—wild and baseless accusations that seemed to spring from the depths of her tortured mind. "You're just like your father," she would hiss, her words like daggers piercing my heart. "You're worthless, just like him." Each accusation, each word of hate, left my body in a state of constant stress, ready to snap at the slightest provocation. I lived in a continual state of fear and insecurity, never knowing when her next outburst would come or what form it would take.

One particular memory seared itself into my mind like a branding iron. I can still feel the rough texture of the grass beneath my hands and the taste of dirt on my lips as I was dragged outside like an animal, a spectacle for the entire neighborhood to witness.

"Look at what you've done!" my mother's voice rang out, dripping with contempt as she yanked me by the hair, dragging me unceremoniously into the yard. "You're nothing but a misbehaving little brat!" I tried to protest, to plead for mercy, but her grip on my hair was like a vice, unyielding and merciless. And then, before I could comprehend what was happening, she forced me down to my knees, pressing my face into the ground. "Eat it!" she demanded, her voice a mixture of anger and triumph. "Eat the grass like the animal you are!" I choked back tears as I complied, each blade of grass a bitter reminder of my perceived inadequacies. I felt the eyes of the neighbors burning into me, their silent judgment, a weight that pressed down upon my already burdened shoulders. Despite the humiliation and shame, there was a fire burning within me—a stubborn refusal to be broken by the cruelty of others. *I'm not an animal,* I thought defiantly, even as the taste of grass filled my mouth and tears streamed down my cheeks. *I'm a survivor, and I will not let this destroy me.*

Though my parents loved me in their fractured way, I recognized that hurt people hurt people, and their wounds were reflections of their own pain. I bore witness to the legacy of suffering passed down through time, a silent testament to the cyclical nature of trauma. Trapped in cycles of abuse perpetuated through history, my parents unwittingly scarred us all. Yet, despite the damage inflicted upon my tender heart, I refused to let bitterness consume my soul, finding within myself the capacity to love and forgive them.

In my desperate attempt to numb emotional pain, I sought solace in the deceptive comfort of sugar, processed foods, fast foods, and refined carbs, consuming until I was sated beyond recognition. Indulging in solitude, I devoured meals hastily and mindlessly, offering no nourishment but instead fueling a destructive cycle. These nutritionally void, dead, low-vibrational foods dulled my senses, further dimming the flicker of hope within me. Fast food, processed carbs, and sweets became addictive crutches, filling the void left by what I lacked in my life and exacerbating physical and mental issues.

THE AFTERMATH

My body carried the scars of anguish well into my teenage years—a viper's tension coiled within my muscles, my once-vibrant features now etched with the stories of inner strife told by cystic acne and nights haunted by insomnia's relentless torment. Hormonal imbalances sent shockwaves of anxiety and depression through my weary soul, transforming each moment into a battleground where sleep remained as elusive as a wisp of smoke, leaving me grappling with shadows in the darkness. Amidst this relentless assault on my physical well-being—gas, bloating, pain, and restless nights—I yearned for deeper nourishment. My gut health spiraled out of control. Ovarian cysts inflicted constant, sharp pain, and excessive bleeding left me feeling depleted and worn. Unbearable fatigue and persistent malaise weighed heavily upon me, adding to the burdens I carried. Through it all, I found myself devoid of confidence, a casualty of my upbringing where self-care was a foreign concept and my mindset sabotaged any potential for growth, nurturing instead a festering self-hate within. My life teetered out of balance on every level, and my soul ached for answers. At times, I stood on the brink of hopelessness as the relentless struggle became the bane of my existence, constantly gnawing at the edges of my sanity while I grappled with the suffocating weight of dark thoughts. There was a light, however, at the end of the tunnel.

THE HEALING

In hindsight, I've come to recognize each of my past experiences served as a stepping stone for personal growth, leading me on a journey to heal myself and offer guidance to others in similar situations. My awakening came one day when I grew weary of feeling perpetually fatigued and unwell. In my quest for transformation and healing, I embarked on a profound exploration: understanding how the food I consumed impacted not just my body but my entire being. It was an enlightening journey, revealing that food isn't merely about satiating hunger; it's about nourishing our souls.

Delving into the concept of high-vibrational living foods, I underwent a paradigm shift that fundamentally changed how I approached nourishment. I realized everything, including food, vibrates with energy, each carrying its unique frequency. High-vibrational foods remain as close to their natural state as possible, bursting with vitality and essential nutrients—fresh, whole ingredients like fruits, vegetables, nuts, seeds, legumes, and whole grains. These foods offer numerous benefits, including fiber for digestive health, antioxidants to combat oxidative stress, and polyphenols for overall wellness.

Transitioning from a diet laden with processed junk to one rich in high-vibrational foods was neither swift nor linear; it was a gradual evolution marked by years of exploration and experimentation. Slowly but surely, I began replacing low-vibrational foods with wholesome, nourishing alternatives, one small change at a time. With each dietary shift, profound transformations unfolded—my blemished face cleared up, my skin radiated with a newfound glow, hormonal imbalances dissipated, chronic pain faded, and restless nights became peaceful. Mental clarity replaced brain fog, guiding me toward new horizons of possibility.

Beyond the physical changes, these dietary shifts ignited a deeper yearning—a hunger for exploration, self-discovery, and the realization of my fullest potential. It was a journey of transformation that transcended the confines of my physical body, touching every aspect of my being and propelling me toward a future filled with promise and possibility.

As my journey with food unfolded, I found my dietary shifts were not merely about physical nourishment; they served as a gateway to deeper healing. I realized the paramount importance of addressing stress, a pervasive obstacle on the path to vitality. Thus, I embraced a multifaceted approach, integrating daily morning and nighttime routines infused with mindfulness, meditation, and yoga. These practices became sacred rituals, offering moments of introspection, release, and renewal. Alongside physical exercise, I carved out spaces for reflection, rewriting the narrative of self-doubt into one of growth and empowerment.

Through the lens of gratitude, I began to perceive the world anew, finding solace and inspiration in the simple joys of life. Yoga became my sanctuary—a space where I could reflect inward, confront negative thought patterns, and cultivate love, compassion, and a growth mindset. Through this practice, I discovered the interconnectedness of mind, body, and spirit and the importance of nurturing each aspect of my being.

As I delved deeper into yoga and other healing practices, I felt compelled to share my journey and newfound wisdom with others. I pursued certifications in yoga teaching, health coaching, and fitness training, recognizing the transformative power of these disciplines to guide others on their paths to wellness. My passion for high-vibrational living also inspired me to explore the culinary arts, becoming a health-focused chef. This holistic approach to healing—integrating nutrition, movement, mindfulness, and self-discovery—formed the foundation of my brand, Free Flowing Health.

At the heart of Free Flowing Health lies the concept of *soul sustenance*—a profound philosophy that extends far beyond mere physical nourishment. It embodies the belief that true well-being encompasses the holistic nourishment of body, mind, and spirit. Through my journey of healing, I came to understand that soul sustenance is about more than just altering dietary habits; it's about embracing a rich blend of love, compassion, and self-care to nurture the soul. It's an awakening to the realization that true vitality stems from attending to every facet of our being. Soul sustenance gently guides us to cultivate profound self-awareness and to heed the gentle whispers of our bodies and hearts. Yet, soul sustenance is not a destination; it's an ongoing journey of growth and discovery. It's an ever-deepening relationship with the nourishment of our entire selves—a sacred connection that intertwines food, body, mind, and spirit. Within these principles lies the essence of Free Flowing Health.

THE TOOL

PRACTICAL STEPS TOWARDS HIGH VIBRATIONAL EATING

Choose Whole, Nutrient-Dense Foods: Opt for foods that are as close to their natural state as possible. Fresh fruits and vegetables, whole grains, nuts, seeds, legumes, and lean proteins are rich in vitamins, minerals, and antioxidants, supporting overall health and vitality.

Prioritize Organic and Locally Sourced Options: Whenever feasible, choose organic produce and locally sourced ingredients. Organic foods are grown without synthetic pesticides and fertilizers, making them cleaner and more environmentally friendly. Locally sourced foods are fresher and often have higher vibrational energy due to their proximity to where they're consumed.

Practice Mindful Eating: Slow down and savor each bite during mealtime. Pay attention to the colors, textures, and flavors of your food. Chew slowly and mindfully, allowing yourself to fully experience the nourishment it provides. Avoid distractions such as screens or multitasking while eating.

Create Sacred Mealtime Rituals: Infuse your mealtime with intention and reverence by creating sacred rituals. This could include saying a prayer or expressing gratitude before eating, setting a beautiful table with candles or flowers, or playing soothing music to create a peaceful ambiance.

Connect with Nature: Whenever possible, eat outdoors or near a window with natural light. Connect with the elements by enjoying meals in nature, such as picnics in the park or meals by the beach. Take a moment to appreciate the beauty and abundance of the natural world as you nourish your body.

EXERCISES AND AFFIRMATIONS FOR DEEPER CONNECTION

Mindful Eating Meditation: Set aside time before a meal to practice mindful eating meditation. Sit comfortably, close your eyes, and take a few deep breaths to center yourself. As you begin to eat, focus on each bite, noticing the sensations in your body and the thoughts that arise. Practice non-judgmental awareness, allowing yourself to fully experience the present moment without attachment or criticism.

Food Blessing Affirmation: Before eating, hold your hands over your food and offer a silent or spoken blessing. Express gratitude for its nourishment, acknowledging the energy and love that went into its creation. Affirmations such as "I am grateful for this food and the nourishment it provides my body, mind, and spirit" can help cultivate a deeper connection with your food.

Journaling Reflections: Keep a journal to record your thoughts and feelings about your relationship with food. Reflect on your eating habits, emotions surrounding food, and any insights or discoveries you make. Use journal prompts such as "What does food mean to me?" or

"How can I cultivate a more loving and intentional relationship with my food?" to deepen your understanding and connection.

Cooking with Intention: Infuse your cooking process with love and intention by setting positive intentions before preparing meals. Visualize your food is filled with nourishing energy and healing vibrations as you chop, stir, and cook—experiment with incorporating herbs, spices, and aromatics known for their healing properties and energetic benefits.

Gratitude Practice: Cultivate a daily gratitude practice centered around food. Take a moment before each meal to express gratitude for the abundance of nourishment in your life, whether it's the food on your plate, the hands that prepared it, or the earth that provided it. Make it a habit to acknowledge and appreciate the blessings of each mealtime.

To hear the audio version of my mindful eating meditation, visit www.freeflowinghealth/mindfuleatingmeditation.

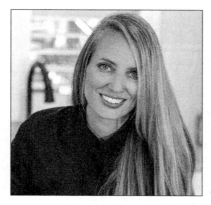

Lisa Brown is a renowned plant-based chef, retreat leader, lifestyle coach, health educator, yoga teacher, personal trainer, podcast host, and visionary founder of Free Flowing Health. With over two decades of dedication, she empowers individuals to transform their lives through healthier lifestyle habits, mindfulness techniques, physical fitness, and high-vibrational eating. Holding a Master's in forensic psychology, Lisa's understanding of human behavior enriches her holistic approach to wellness.

Born and raised in the vibrant streets of New York City, Lisa experienced firsthand the toll of a fast-paced lifestyle. Juggling full-time EMT work with college studies led to severe health issues, including a debilitating back injury, hormonal imbalances, and emotional turmoil from past trauma. However, her journey took a profound turn when she embraced yoga for physical rehabilitation, catalyzing pivotal changes to her lifestyle, diet, and mindset.

Armed with her personal triumph over adversity, Lisa's passion for healthy living blossomed, igniting a profound desire to serve others. With multiple yoga certifications from prestigious institutions, specialized training in trauma-informed yoga and youth at risk, Lisa has accumulated nearly 1,000 hours of study. Additionally, she is a certified health coach from the Institute for Integrative Nutrition and a NASM-certified personal trainer. Lisa received her culinary education from the Natural Gourmet Institute in NYC.

Today, she seamlessly integrates her expertise as a chef, coach, and educator to guide individuals worldwide toward greater levels of health, happiness, and harmony.

Explore the path to vibrant living by contacting Lisa and the Free Flowing Health team for personalized chef services and lifestyle coaching at www.freeflowinghealth.com.

CHAPTER 20

KINTSUGI
THE GOLDEN LINES OF INTEGRATIVE HEALING ARTS

ALCHEMIZING SACRED SCARS INTO SERENITY AND JOY FOR RADIANT REBIRTH

Nydia Laysa Stone, Somatic Healing Artist, Therapist, Coach

CRACKED OPEN

We see the world not as it is, but as we are

with eyes of our wounded hearts

and wombs

Our rough and broken boundaries

from rough and broken hands

lost

in unchecked desire

May love become the artist

to sand my jagged edges smooth

Let fires of resilience burn!

Bright gleaming Gold flow in my scars

to do its dance of alchemy

and crack me into Beauty

Now, I can see my world again

the way

I am

Nydia Laysa Stone

**WHAT IF YOU AREN'T BROKEN
BUT A HUMAN MASTERPIECE OF ART
IN CONSTANT CREATION?**

MY STORY

TRACING SCARS BEYOND THE SMILES

All of me wants to pull back, run, scream, and hide!

But my fingertips are still exploring these rough, dried-up cracks and craters, tracing broken edges and fragmentations—like deep, sinister scars on my skin.

Vague images flash through me—a strong sense of unease stirring—first whispers of something shifting in my core, spreading like delicate spiderwebs.

My stomach contracts into a fist of iron, and nausea rises, consuming me.

I gasp to catch and steady my breath.

"You're okay?" Anna studies me, concerned, scanning my skin, encrusted with dried mud—reminiscent of leprosy.

We joined a gathering in Goa, where I intended to sell some of my artwork.

I'm 19.

Living in India between the peace, love, and sexual liberation of the hippie revolution, ashrams, and sadhus, I study therapy, Yoga, meditation, Tantra, and life!

We camp at the river, and my slipping in the mud had just initiated a mudbath with lots of jokes and laughter.

Smelling this rich, nourishing earth, I wrapped it all around me like armor, a magician's cape—I'm invisible!—my inner medicine woman, merging into Gaia.

Under the blazing Indian sun, the mud dries quickly; mesmerized, I observe the landscape on my body transform: It cracks open, separates into fragments, and crumbles off, forming deep crevices, like wounds, holding ancient secrets and mysteries, dark as graves at midnight. My spirit grows heavy.

Completely absorbed, I start tracing these hardened lines, feeling the tugging and pulling of energetic strings and subtle connections between the "scars" under my fingertips and the woundings of my soul, the brand marks of my ancestral and collective heritage—in my heart, my womb, my yoni-flower.

I try to smile at Anna, my pulse drumming hard against my ribs.

Beneath the smiles and laughter, though—I sense the danger.

BLACK HOLES AND HUNGRY GHOSTS

I'm courageous, travel, and live alone in foreign countries, but there are moments when I feel these bottomless, terrifying hollow spaces below; there are rips and tears, sudden black holes I fall through into this void of lack and neediness—getting lost in time and space, in visions, overwhelming emotions, unpredictable responses, and reactions. I'm escaping, searching for security.

My body doesn't seem a safe place.

I've always managed to struggle my way back up and out. I don't want to see!

But I know, right here and now: *It's time!*

I can't keep ignoring the knocking and banging against these guarded portals, like passage rites into my dark, moist alleyways, the labyrinth of my inner catacombs, where my monsters and hungry ghosts hang out.

Starkly, I see the gates in front of me:

Do I dare turn the key?

These dreary stairways I have staggered down before! Screams of pain and anguish, echoing in the vault.

I still smell these fears of torture and fire—my lineage!

Dizziness grabs me—I call out for protection from my goddesses, my guides, and guardians!

Soft angel wings embrace my anxious heart. I breathe, take another step

—and trace another dried-out line on my skin.

I feel as part of this earth on my body, nourished, embraced, and held by the elements; immersed, belonging, and intertwining with something bigger than me—and begin honoring, cherishing, even loving these lines, fragmentations, and imperfections of myself.

Without further thought or wondering, I retrieve my art supplies, pouring paints into these scars and crevices.

First, my favorites: *I am water!*

In shimmering rivers of turquoise blues and greens, they flow down my breasts, my belly, bringing life into the dried-out deserts of my inner realms.

Abruptly, panic kicks in, and my alarm system triggers!

LEAP OF FAITH: DEFYING VICTIMIZING SHAME INTO DIGNITY

I've been familiar with these sudden "journeys" since childhood:

My sight blurring—a flood of images, sensations, and emotions tumbling and swirling, sweeping me out of the present moment like a tsunami!

I see these fat red fingers on my belly, crushing the flowers on my dress;

an 'uncle' giving me horsey rides, rocking my reluctant 5-year-old body on his knees.

Hush. Don't lie! Can't tell anyone! Dirty! Secret!

These disgusting bluish swollen lips—always glistening, leaving dewy marks on my skin!

Time warp!

I am nine . . .

. . . this big boy holding me down with his heavy, slippery body—his friends cheering!

Scratchy grass against my bare back, my cheek wet from his forced kisses!

Feeling helpless, weak, humiliated—I finally struggle free, escape!

Have to get high—above the world, above things!

Height has always held safety for me, a change of perspective.

Distress and shame drive me towards the trees, my friends and allies!

But they are too small here!

Desperate, I climb into the refuge of the ten-meter tower above the pool.

The agonizing cheering of his friends still echoing in my ears, I frantically rub and scratch my cheek until my blood runs red onto my hands.

Instinctively, I decide on an act of bravery to reclaim my dignity and self-respect!

Singing my 'Dragon Songs' to encourage myself, I step out onto the oscillating, swaying diving board, the water below frighteningly distant!

I'm a good swimmer, but I have never dared to jump from this tower.

My toes curl around the edge of the long, quivering plank; I swallow hard, fill my lungs with air, and bend my knees:

With a scream of victory, I catapult myself off the board!

In mid-flight, I already spin into a different memory.

I am 13 . . .

Some small festival.

This young artist is painting my back. We are joking— until the energy shifts and his hands start moving with different intentions. I freeze! Like a deer trapped in the headlights of a car, paralyzed by this wave of unchecked masculine desire.

I'm this little girl again. *Dirty secrets, can't tell anyone. Blood on my cheeks.*

But then my inner warrior erupts in violent rage. I scream, spit, and bite and can't stop—just can't stop!

PASSAGE RITES: HEALING THE WOUNDED FEMININE

I wander, lost, adrift between times and events, trembling and shaking.

A woman's soft voice reaches me through the haze; I can't understand the words but hear and sense the love. All my fury dissipates and vanishes, and I sink into the embrace of this voice like the desperate child, the wounded woman I am.

She sings and cradles me all night, anchoring me with my breath, as my emotions swing wildly between weeping helplessly in deepest, curled-up despair and shame and my outbursts of frenzy, maddening fury and aggression.

Silvery moonlight falls on my exhausted body through the open smoke flaps.

"Your tipi is like a cathedral."

The flickering flames reflect in her deep, knowing eyes; she smells like forest, amber, and something powerful, mystical. Her long dark hair caresses my heart while she bends over to tend to her fire; a sense of homecoming spreads in me.

She feels like a mother, grandmother, sister—a wise druidess, guiding me through these dark, turbulent seas with her presence and voice, her humming hands on my body.

"How can I become like you?" She studies me for a while.

"You are already, my daughter. They found and called you. Just keep walking and listening."

Her answer is cryptic but something within me understands.

REMEMBRANCE: THE BODY HOLDS THE HEALING

"What happened then, Eliza?"

"You kicked and bit him, pulled his hair."

"He didn't ask permission!"

"All is good now. Breathe like I showed you, sweetheart."

Slowly, my racing heartbeat calms down again.

"Do you think I'm crazy, like mad or schizophrenic?"

She lets out a small laugh.

"No, you are not insane. You must have been hurt deeply. And your body retains the memory. All is etched into our bodies. But the body also holds the healing. You can trust the wisdom of your body, always!"

I have to remember this.

COMING HOME INTO THE BODY

At the river, chills of unease run down my spine; I feel the painful pull of fine hair rising on end, caught in the hardened earth on my skin.

My body in panic—my mind, in distress, still eagerly insists on clinging to the illusionary safety and outdated framework of limitations and fears.

I must remember—trust the body!

I'm terrified! but entranced by the powerful flow of energy pulsing through me now. With a shaky, trembling breath, I gaze back down at these cracks and fragmentations, the blue rivers slowly streaming down my belly, between my thighs.

My seat of power!

"Own it!" I hear Eliza say.

METAMORPHOSIS: LET THE MAGIC HAPPEN

Remember who you are! whisper my ancestors.

Driven by impulse, I reach for my colors again:

Some more greens and blues!

I'm a storyteller, a Dreamweaver flying my dragons, a skydancer, Dakini!

Graceful, light-footed, light-hearted, powerful!

Fiery reds and orange!

Sacred flames of Kali Ma—the phoenix rising!

Some feathers now!

Quetzalcoatl—feathered serpent dragon wisdom!

Condor! Colibri—I'm an air being!

And the gold!

I fill the rough edges with golden compassion for this brave little warrior girl— honor her pain, fears, and her courage. By illuminating her sacred wounds, I make them mine, own them in their radiant beauty—**amor fati!**

I highlight them with glitter and mother of pearl—my womb, my soul, and body, a gleaming, sparkling testimony of my love, resilience, and victory!

DIVINE BRUSHSTROKES INTO EMOTIONAL FREEDOM

And here comes this moment when I just let it all go—fully surrender to the process, cut the chains of my need to control, entrusting the reins into the Divine hands and remembrance of my ancient inner knowings, the somatic intelligence of my body, the innate wisdom of my womb— and let this intuition guide me, my wide open heart leading the way.

The whispers and songlines of my guardians and ancestors embrace my hands, leading my playful brush, layering paints, and weaving feathers and pearls into my braids.

Mama Jaguar walks fearlessly through the darkest corners of my catacombs, setting free my oldest demons.

Kali's purifying fires consume outdated versions, beliefs, traces of muck, and traumatic residues. My angels shine the light of eternal, unconditional love into my inner world, my soul.

They bestow their blessings of Grace on these fractures, lesions of all my lifetimes, and dismantle the witch wound and all collective trauma since Lilith ate the apple.

They plow my inner soils, so I can plant my fresh new seeds of joy and sovereignty deep within my fertile grounds.

They unblock the channels, allowing the healing waters to flow freely and nurture these seedlings with their pure, sparkling elixirs and divine nectars of Amrita, weaving an emboldened, luminous fabric with the touch of golden compassion, a perfect symbiosis of body, emotion, and spirit ... all flowing in harmony.

Once I give my permission, they all know what to do, where to mend, caress, tear apart, and rebuild, all working hand in hand on this 'beautiful destruction' of my old forms, beliefs, and programming.

I just need to trust and get out of the way!

EMPOWERED EMBODIMENT EXPRESSION

Painting and decorating, I keep honoring my body temple. Graceful serenity rises— pride!

I feel liberated, free, whole, at peace—untouchable.

On my walk back to the market, the scars on my earthy skin are glowing, radiating with blues, golds, and feathers—sparkling joy!

My transformation is mirrored in the gazing eyes of others.

Takashi, a Japanese student, marvels at me with surprise and bewilderment.

"You look like an ancient warrior Goddess, like a living Kintsugi sculpture!"

My tool is born!

Takashi Itohara—my gratitude! Wherever you are in the world!

I'm still small, but brave to meet my fears and monsters, alchemizing my wounds and imperfections into golden paths of expansion, serenity, and sensual liberation.

Until today, I'm shaping, shifting, and crafting on the ever-evolving canvas of my personal magnum opus, integrating and illuminating all my flaws, a human masterpiece in constant creation and renewal, forever changing and transforming. Forever unique and magnificent!

MIRACLES ARE SIMPLY A SHIFT IN PERCEPTION

Do you ever dream of wielding a magic wand to paint your life's canvas with more vibrancy, freedom, and lightheartedness?

More alignment, adventure, love, and laughter – wouldn't that be marvelous?

My first encounter with Kintsugi mindset at this river in Goa was an intuitive somatic exploration, wholly guided by my inner knowing.

My willingness and courage to trust this voice and the Divine process shifted my restricted perception, beliefs, and conditioning, opened me up to beauty, wonder, and **different choices**, and thus rewired my nervous system.

THE 'OPEN SESAME' TO RESET

As Takashi introduced me to this fascinating Japanese concept of Fine Arts and philosophy, where the brokenness of objects—or humans—is adorned with gold, embodying the beauty within imperfection, I was inspired and immediately fell under the spell of these 'Golden Lines', integrated them into my life, downloading and weaving these codes into my matrix.

In my sessions and retreats, both in art and as a therapist, I offer and employ Kintsugi as a transformative code—a magical 'Open Sesame'—revealing boundless horizons and depth for a profound reset, by alchemizing the torn, shattered, and unspeakable into radiant serenity and joy.

Here is a first experience for you!

THE TOOL

KINTSUGI - GOLDEN CODES TO REWIRE AND SHINE

Let Your Body Be Your Compass

Trust your innate wisdom and somatic intelligence.

Create Sacred Space

Call in Higher Guidance and protection.

Ground

Drop into your breath, shake, sound (activate the vagus nerve).

Set Your Intention: Be Brave, Clear, Creative

Give your body-mind positive directions, impulses, and focus.

Open pathways to rewire your nervous system.

I am Safe and Guarded
Install somatic anchors before the session:
breath, mudra, touch, color, sound, tapping.

Activate Agni—Flames of Transformation
Create heat: move and rub hands, feet, and body.

SHALL WE START THE ADVENTURE?
1. Choose and Prepare your Body-Canvas: A, B, or C?
A) Choose a photo or draw outlines of your body on paper.
This can be a small or life-size body map.
B) Choose a symbolic object.
Winged Pegasus? Angel? Shell, root, something representing your body.
C) Choose your physical body as a living canvas.
This is a deeply somatic experience. Beware of triggers.

BODY PAINTING RITUAL WITH EARTH, CLAY, OR PAINT.
While it dries and cracks, scratch marks, symbols, scars, and lines into
the clay.
Let my story inspire your process.

FEEL – SEE – LET IT BE
Once you've chosen your canvas:
2. Feel into all the questions of your INNER LANDSCAPE (see below).
3. Transmute and mark your sensations and emotions on your chosen body canvas.
Find a symbol, image, sound, gesture, or word to represent
your feelings.

Write, draw, tear holes, paint, wrinkle, scratch, decorate, beautify...

All are welcome.

Don't overthink this process! Stay present. Let intuition guide you!

Observe with empathy and childlike curiosity.

WITNESS WITHOUT ANALYZING, JUDGING, OR FINDING SOLUTIONS.

4. Feel into the fragmentations, the shattered, your scars.

Paint or sculpt these scars onto your body-canvas.

5. Tear or cut up the photo/paper along these scars.

Or break the object (like the wing of the pegasus).

6. Connect with these scars on your canvas—let them be seen.

If it feels safe, hold your hands on these scars of your physical body.

Sit with the sensations of your experiences.

They are your past, your story. They brought you here.

Can you accept that they are part of your life and beauty?

REMEMBER YOUR INTENTION!

Do you allow these events and sufferings to define you?

Do you want to heal, write your own script, and move on?

Rewire or rebirth?

It's a decision. It requires courage.

You are the heroine of your journey!

LOVE AND HONOR – LET GO AND GROW

7. Embrace your imperfections and trauma.

Honor your courage to walk your healing path!

Lovingly re-assemble your fragments.

Glue the broken pieces onto a bigger carton, leaving spaces between the scars. Create a new form and identity of yourself.

Write, paint, and illuminate instead of hiding.

Honor these scars of pain and grief.

Fill them with symbols, colors, and feathers!

With love, light, and golden compassion.

Step consciously into joy!

Celebrate yourself!

Let the magic happen!

SHINE!

* * *

INNER LANDSCAPE (from above)

Send your breath, your loving awareness, and attention to all areas of your physical body.

LET IT RISE. Explore and listen.

If anxiety emerges, drop back into your breath.

Anchor and confirm yourself: "I am safe."

Where in your body do you feel disconnected, heavy, tight, hardened, fearful, sad, empty, blocked, fragmented, torn, shattered, separated, dirty, unworthy, strange, outside the norm?

Which body areas seem inaccessible, like they don't belong to you?

Who do they belong to—your husband, children, family, society, past events, your beliefs?

How would you describe the INNER LANDSCAPE of your different body areas?

Textures, colors, mountains, valleys, desert, forest, ocean, rivers:

Still or windy, stormy, cold, hot, moist, dry, fertile, burning.

Which sounds, words, or emotions come up while you're traveling through your inner landscapes?

Where in your body reside hope, love, trust, dreams, joy, pleasure, or freedom?

Where is your seat of power? Does it feel activated, alive?

Detect spaces full of life force and energy!

Write, paint, sculpt, destroy, mend, and decorate your healing map.

* * *

Find more Free guidance, meditations & practices

Free challenges and integrations

Info about all Immersive Global Retreats

Tantric Yoni Arts & Womb Wisdom

AUDIO guidance for TOOL and chapter on
https://www.healingartsbynydia.com/kintsugi

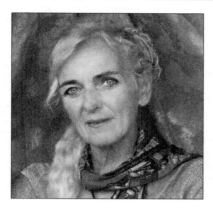

Nydia Laysa Stone, Somatic Therapist, Life Transition Coach, Bestselling Author, New Earth Visionary and Healing Artist.

Miracles are just a shift in perception

Let's explore your awakening path toward joyful, sensual living and your journey of healing and transformation. Reclaim your power and authenticity through Tantric Embodiment practices, Vision Quest, Shamanic Ceremonies, integrating Yoga, art, and neuroscience. Nydia is an experienced master teacher of the Healing Arts, Violet Flame, Egyptian Sekhem energy, Reiki, and worldwide light code activations, Yoga, Tantra, breathwork, dynamic meditations, dance & art expression, soul retrieval, and the Rites of the Munay Ki.

She is passionate about movement in all its forms, overcoming stagnation and catalyzing change toward empowered expansion.

Her signature REWILDING Retreats for Women are transformative experiences: cultural and spiritual immersions in the world's most significant high-vibrational locations, including Egypt, Peru, India, Bali, Fiji, Greece, and the Caribbean Islands – Nydia's chosen 'homelands'. For over 35 years, she has lived, studied, and worked as a global nomad in these inspiring environments.

Based on Tantric and sensual explorations, as well as Somatic embodiment practices, Nydia's curated sessions and retreats will connect you to your inner knowing, innate womb wisdom, and ancestral lineage to awaken the Wild Wise Warrior and Medicine Woman within.

Nydia will guide you through vision quests and passage rites, igniting your life transitions to find alignment, purpose, and focus and initiate sacred shifts and your soulful metamorphosis toward the liberated, joyful, and heart-centered life of your dreams!

You can often find Nydia in canyons, climbing on a rope over waterfalls, barefoot, dancing Salsa on tropical beaches, singing around a campfire, or cuddling some furry friend. She loves elephants, jaguars, and mangoes.

Nydia communicates fluently in English, German, French, and Spanish.

Work with Nydia:

Linktree: https://www.linktr.ee/healingartsbynydia

Instagram: https://www.instagram.com/nydia.laysa.stone/

https://www.instagram.com/healingartsbynydia/

Facebook: https://www.facebook.com/nydialaysastone

Website: https://www.HealingArtsbyNydia.com

CHAPTER 21

AROMA ORACLES

BREAKING THROUGH THE STATIC

Charlotte Warn

MY STORY

The sun was shining bright and warm through the sliding glass door. His hard penis touching my hand was something I'd never experienced. I was four.

"Don't tell anyone, or we'll both be in trouble," he said. This was my earliest memory of the many traumatic encounters I endured growing up. This continued with this person until I was nine years old. I grew up with a lot of anger in my heart. Later in life, I felt completely cheated of my childhood. I watched many of my friends have a sense of freedom and innocence in their hearts, whereas I felt guarded, scared, confused, and angry. I was always in trouble or doing something wrong. I was always pretending to be someone other than myself. I was masking who I truly was. I felt too ashamed and thought people would not like me for who I am, someone with such nasty secrets.

As I got older, I lost my virginity to rape. *What the fuck?!* All trust was gone. I had a few more encounters after that and felt I was never understood by anyone. I strived to find comfort in the indie culture. I masked in many ways. I was a punk rock kid with an electric blue mohawk; I followed the Grateful Dead, smoked a lot of pot, and did a lot of psychedelics. I still felt so guarded and imprisoned. And honestly, I thought sex equaled love. *Wrong!*

My father lived in Sedona, Arizona. When I turned 21, he challenged me to stay put for one solid year. I never lived in one place for very long. I attended four different high schools. No, my parents were not in the military.

"I bet you can't stay still for 12 months," my dad said. Oh, how I loved a good challenge. My father, being a spiritual man and a healer, knew my language and how to help me find myself. I stayed put, and to this day, I still call that time in my life my spiritual boot camp. There's something really healing in nature, especially among those sacred red rocks. I simply got lost for days all by myself, and I cherished every moment. My father was a wonderful teacher for me, even more so after his passing in 2017. He taught me about meditation and energy at a very young age. That certainly came in handy. For that, I'm so grateful. During traumas, I could simply check out and basically leave my body with the tools of meditation that were taught to me. Later in life, these survival tactics ceased to work. I thought I was going crazy. I then realized Source was giving me the opportunity to fully heal from these traumas and no longer feel the need to mask in life and build true friendships and intimate relationships.

My mother is a very linear woman who is amazing at finances and business. How blessed am I to have had both sides of the coin in my pockets in terms of influence? I'm truly grateful. The two of them divorced when I was five years old.

They say time heals all wounds. I call bullshit on that. However, I feel time gifts us with many experiences, a plethora of perspectives, and a multitude of paradigms. With that being said, I feel the saying ought to be, "Time grants us the opportunities to transcend all wounds." Being a survivor of trauma, for me—in the world according to Charli (my nickname)—some or perhaps all traumas never truly go away. But I've discovered these traumas are mine. They are part of the very make-up of who I am. I'd be someone else without these experiences. Through my recovery, I feel very called to share some of the ways I've healed and thrived.

I used to be able to simply check out. When I was reminded of a trauma or triggered, I could simply check out, become someone else, stuff those emotions down, and push them away. I liked to get silly, crack sarcastic jokes, or simply blow it off. Like I had mentioned, there came a time when those tactics no longer worked. I became very depressed and slightly suicidal. Source was not giving me an out. It was time to grow, expand, transcend (whatever you wanna call it). I could no longer walk that path, and it was time for a change.

I went to therapy and tried to hash it all out. This wasn't for me. I think therapy is great and extremely helpful. But it left me feeling very raw and extremely vulnerable, and it all felt quite dramatic. I wanted results. *Let's just be done with it.* I didn't want to walk through all the trauma over and over again. I found it very draining. My brain just doesn't work that way. However, I know it's truly helpful for others, and that's all that matters.

I became a massage therapist in 1990. This was so healing for me. Massage is a safe place to be touched, and I wanted to be able to offer that to others. Many of my clients were trauma survivors as well. I then discovered essential oils. Now, I felt I was on to something. I loved good-smelling aromas! I smell them all of the time, wear them, and diffuse them. I became certified in The Raindrop Technique in 2009; this, too, was very healing and helpful. I discovered that if I smelled oils often on good days, when I had tough days, smelling oils automatically took my mind to the good days. I slowly created new synapses. Oh, what a game-changer!

Over time, I combined much of my training and certifications and developed Aroma Oracles to help others heal.

THE TOOL

Aroma Oracles. What the heck is that?

What would life be like if we actually woke up in the morning and felt love in our hearts for ourselves and the life we are living?

I got the calling to combine many of my certifications, experiences, intuition, and knowledge into one basket. I like to say I help folks navigate through their static. Man, we all got it! We all have baggage, trials, tribulations, secrets, and disharmonies.

I use many decks of oracle cards, essential oils, and other modalities to tap into those roadblocks. These tools can lend insights to alternative perspectives. I love to use pure essential oils in all of my sessions. When inhaled, essential oils affect the olfactory senses—your smell sense. The molecules then affect the limbic region of the brain. This is where your memories and emotions are stored. The job of essential oils is to clean off the receptor sites of our cells so they communicate better with one another. How cool is that? So, when you inhale a pure essential oil, you can then begin to think clearer, just like that! It does not get much easier.

The Oracle cards are a tool to help me feel what's happening with you. I'm not a fortune teller or a prophet. I simply help guide you through the static to receive new perspectives within yourself. In other words, I like to help empower folks. Nobody knows you better than you! Only you truly know what's best for you and what you actually want. Sometimes, that's the hardest part of growing.

You might ask yourself: *What is it that I want?*

Let's try this out. This is a quick Aroma Reset, one of the many modalities I offer and one of the easiest. This is something you can do numerous times a day if needed. Let's say you've had a really rough day. Everything is pushing your buttons, and you just can't seem to shake it. Pause. Let's do a quick scan. If you were to explain what you're feeling in that very moment in one basic feeling word (yes, one basic feeling word), what would that word be? Perhaps angry, sad, mad, afraid? One basic feeling word. Got it? Now, let's do a body scan. Take a deep breath and imagine that feeling as a scanner moving over your entire body like a beam of light. Where in your body are you physically feeling this emotion or feeling? Sometimes, it may be tricky, but one body part may come to your thoughts. Acknowledge this. Now, you have your one feeling word and where you feel this in your body.

I invite you to take out an essential oil. I love to use Young Living Essential Oils, as I know they're pure and unadulterated, and I don't get the same results using other brands. It doesn't really matter which essential oil aroma; however, citrus oils are great to use when you're feeling blue—like lemon, tangerine, grapefruit, bergamot, or citrus fresh. Floral oils are good for when you're feeling angry or heated—like lavender, geranium, rose, and a wonderful blend called Peace and Calming.

Please know there are no rules to this, and you're welcome to use any essential oil aroma that seems inviting. Now, go ahead and drop one drop of the essential oil onto one of your palms, rub your hands together, and cup your hands over your nose. I like to call this a scent tent. Inhale and simply notice what you're noticing. No need to judge or analyze. Simply take notice; observe. Has your emotion shifted, escalated, dissolved? Have you received any ideas or revelations, or do you feel you need a little something more or need to have a friend simply listen? Sometimes, someone to simply bear witness to you is incredibly powerful and comforting.

In the next step, we can move further along and go a bit deeper with other modalities, like the Aroma Freedom Technique, to help transcend blocks, wounds, or traumas. This is a great tool I offer to gently shift awareness away from negative thoughts, feelings, and memories and to initiate a positive outlook and attitude. This tool was a game changer for me and my personal growth! I wish I'd known about it earlier. It would've saved me decades of self-loathing and expensive therapy sessions. However, I'm now astonishingly grateful for every moment. I now know that all my experiences were a language I needed to experience to bring me to the gifts I'm now privileged to share with others.

Back to the Aroma Freedom Technique, created by Dr. Benjamin Perkus. Aroma Freedom is an entirely new way of using pure essential oils, combined with proven psychological principles, to quickly and gently dissolve the negative thoughts, feelings, and memories that hold us back from reaching our dreams. It uses the principle of memory reconsolidation, which has been studied by modern neuroscience as the natural way that the brain updates learning and prediction.

According to Dr. Perkus, "I discovered that holding the four primary aspects of consciousness together at the same time (feeling, thought, sensation, and imagination) while smelling specific essential oils had the effect of "dissolving" the memory/emotion complex, and allowed the person to become free from the effects of negative experiences from the past. I further discovered that the same process can be used when considering current experiences and future imaginings. We now have techniques that are wonderful for goal setting, stress reduction, relief from painful memories, and overall mental and emotional balance."

I truly love what I do, working with my clients and witnessing their new awareness and breakthroughs. I have one client whom I met in a time of great turmoil in her life and on the verge of divorce. She came for readings, the Aroma Freedom Technique, and a few sessions of Dream Building. She gained new perspectives and possibilities for herself. I helped her create a blueprint to achieve more harmony. She now has a renewed and refreshed relationship with her husband and is now working at her dream job.

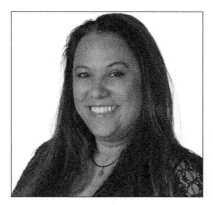

Charlotte Warn, the visionary behind Aroma Oracles is the torchbearer of a lineage steeped in spiritual healing traditions. With a rich tapestry of over three decades in the healing arts, she continues to honor the legacy of her late father, who was a renowned psychic surgeon. Her unwavering commitment lies in guiding individuals towards self-transformation, awakening their intuitive wisdom, and leading profoundly fulfilling lives.

In 1990, Charlotte embarked on her holistic journey by attending massage school, a pivotal moment that opened the doors to her exploration of the wellness realm. Her intuitive gifts flourished amidst the breathtaking red rocks of Sedona, Arizona, where she settled in 1992. Since then, she's been an ardent student of self-wisdom and personal expansion.

Throughout her journey, Charlotte has acquired numerous certifications across a diverse spectrum of modalities. These skills enable her to craft tailored and distinctive healing experiences for everyone she assists.

Beyond her mastery of healing modalities, Charlotte also conducts captivating workshops, offers transformative life coaching, and orchestrates expansive retreats on both national and international stages.

Charlotte's core belief centers on the idea that everyone possesses a soul's purpose. Her passion lies in empowering individuals to design and manifest lives in perfect harmony with their unique path, granting them the opportunity to live lives they genuinely adore.

Connect with Charlotte:

Facebook and Instagram @AromaOracles.
Website: www.charlottewarn.com
Email: aromaoracles@gmail.com
Some of Charlotte's favorite essential oils:
https://bit.ly/Charlotte_Favorite

CHAPTER 22

REFLECTION OF YOUR GIFT

THE MIRROR OF REALIZATION

T. Brandon Russ, Medium, Astrologer, Life Coach

MY STORY

Imagine your whole life saying the wrong thing in the worst situations. Yep, that's me. It took me years to understand that my sometimes-gregarious nature, boundless energy, and unrelenting positivity were a calling card with purpose on my journey. I learned how to help others with my quirky gift.

After spending years taking development classes, I was more than ready to step out on my own. I was appreciative of the gift, but I still hadn't gotten it down to a science. I tried to take this magical gift of mine and figure it out. It led me to multiple pursuits, becoming a spiritual life coach, Reiki master teacher, and the study of astrology.

My first astrology teacher was old school and hard-core with the tools of calculation. He only allowed 'green sheets' of the sky, and you needed the discipline of drawing each planet and asteroid by its symbol. The lines needed to be meticulously calculated to specific ratios and angles to project the influence of the blah, blah blah… I appreciated the knowledge but only wanted to understand why I was built the way I am.

I spent time figuring myself out, believing that astrology was a primer code of my strengths and weaknesses and where I was meant to focus my energy. I think of astrology as your personal SWOT analysis of self. I think I figured it out, or at least after significant study time, I realized what I was good at and what my challenges might be. It brings me back to that moment when a teacher said to me, "You are learning this for a reason. You might not know it yet, but you will know it when you get there." I realized I was learning all these disciplines and astrology because they held some destiny and personality traits that people could identify in their path. Answering, "Why am I like this?" Spirit began to show me astrology in readings when people needed to understand their paths and patterns.

* * *

I greeted Grace as she sat down in the oversized Barca lounger the chiropractor had in the office I rented on Saturdays.

"I'm sorry, I'm a little nervous. I've never done this before." She said with an elegance that carried her name.

"Me either," I said with a humorous quip. Sarcasm as a tool is timely when you have been an active full-time medium for over 12 years having over 20,000 readings experience.

I walked through the routine of connections. My guides, my angels, my everything. She bowed her head as if she was in church.

I connected with her prim and proper grandmother. The tea-totaling ethical matriarch who blended the family name with a socialite edge from an age that emerged aristocrats stepped through. The gown she wore as she walked into my mind's eye was stunning. Her pearls were designed to fit properly on the doily lace with embroidered embellishments. Her hair was held up in a bun without a single stray. It accentuated her pearls around the neckline. At the center of the necklace was a cameo pendant lying down on her chest in perfect symmetry. It was meant to stand out and be seen.

When Spirit presents itself, it comes in two primary ways: figurative and literal. The figurative is often metaphoric and may have many meanings. For example, they may show a stop sign, which could mean eight sides, red, or "stop." There are avenues in which it can go, almost like a choose-your-own-adventure in messages. The metaphors shown are just like the charade game it implies; it could be this or that. They are often colloquial guidance or opinions of a situation for the person I'm connecting with in the reading. This is a proxy evidential point and only proves a connection if you believe it is a message. The literal, however, is more direct and often undeniable. In a sense, it provides the confidence someone needs to prove a valid connection. Presenting and representing something tangible. In this case, the cameo was specific and had meaning to her instantly.

"Yes, yes!" she exclaimed. "That is her, most definitely her! She raised me; she was my everything." She was relieved that this experience was now 'real.' She had heard so many speculative stories. This was undeniably her grandmother, her namesake. She pulled out the cameo from her purse. "This is her, and this is me." The carved ivory against the coral oval was a striking resemblance to Grace and her grandmother.

I felt like Grace had fallen far from this well-to-do life her grandmother was showing me. She wanted me to help her.

"April 28th, the morning. The overnight. Evelyn says I am cold; you are okay." I spouted the channel I was tuned into. I saw her chart; I could see Grace's potential. Her flaws. The lessons that she was born into astrologically. I often have no idea what I'm saying, at least in context. That is the magic of sitting with a medium. They shouldn't know what they see. The lack of context in the initial moments is critical to authenticity. The details always come next. But I needed to reassure Grace.

"Th-That's my mother, Evelyn. She was an ice queen, and that's my birthday," she said exhaling as if to get it all out in the air. It was as if we were in a confessional, and the energy was flowing towards forgiveness.

Mediums are really scientists at the end of the day. They are inundated with information and begin to problem-solve and ultimately, they are trying to find validation for what they are seeing, sensing, etc. I began to tell Grace what her grandmother and mother had shown me.

"You are the center of your own attention." I began to tread softly but directly with my words. I was shown a two-way mirror.

She's vain, she's self-centered, and she self-sabotages as a matter of operation. She's not married, she's alone and she's desperate now as she has run through her inheritance, is single, and broke because of bad pre-nuptial agreements and Veruca Salt lifestyle. She had no other choice than to change.

"Your grandmother shows me, you are alone and it's part them and part you." She listened intently not to interrupt. "She's reassuring you that the money will be okay because it's just money." Grace scoffed at the notion. "Well, tell her, she spent plenty of money on her own and that could have helped me now if she didn't."

Her demeanor broke as her thoughts were fragmented and often scattered.

"I didn't do anything that someone else wouldn't have done," she continued.

Sun Conjunct Mercury Conjunct Jupiter, all in Taurus. First house all the way. All about her. No one above her; no use for anyone but. . .

"Jack was different, a true love," I said specifically.

"What about Jack?" she looked at me side-eyed. She reached down to her purse and pulled it closer to her. "He was my ex-husband. And I'm not sure he was a true love. He wasn't faithful."

"He might not have been, but he knows you weren't either." Her face was drawn and flushed all at once. "Sometimes we connect with people Karmatically. They have a purpose and a lesson for us in our path. We can turn them into a villain in our story or we can be grateful they were the messenger of the lesson we needed."

"He was mean to me," she pouted like a child who was told no. "I'm not going to talk about him."

"Your grandmother is talking about the ice cream date and the cameo you wore. Skinny 8, pineapple, and down at the shoreline. Your sweater. Back to the car, and he gave you his jacket." I sat in the moment, in a trance to connect with my clairvoyant ability.

"I guess it wasn't all bad. He asked me about the pendant, and we talked about her all night." She spoke with clarity. She felt empowered, too.

I knew she was comfortable here, controlling the dialog and being able to tell the story. *Her grandmother brought Jack and Grace together.*

"He was wonderful at first. His eyes, his hair. Rugged. Sophisticated and a powerhouse of energy. We talked every day from that moment until it was over. He changed. I found out who he was over time." Her voice tailed away as if to have her visions of what happened next in the five-year relationship.

"She shows me the wedding on the cliff, the ice sculptures, and the hundreds of people," I was direct and to the point. This is how she likes her conversations, appealing to that Mercury in Taurus.

Her grandmother had helped the two of them to meet. Jack was everything she needed and a perfect compliment to her. He had patience and success. Their nodes lined up, their Moon and Venus complimented. They were beyond Karmatic partners, they were indeed **soulmates**.

"He's a one, and you're a seven," I quipped. "Your life path numbers."

"How do you know all this?" she asked, doing the math in her head. "He is a life path one."

"Your grandmother told me."

The compatibility of life paths one and seven is strong. They complement one another when it comes to connection, spiritual life, and dreams and goals. The strength of life path one compliments the weakness of the seven and vice versa.

She looked down at the table and reached for a tissue. A seal had been broken, and she wasn't able to hold back. "He hurt me," she gaslighted the narrative, trying to convince me that she was in an abusive relationship.

Jupiter in conjunction with the Sun First house. Tendency to over-inflate everything.

"It was the things he said, not only what he did. He didn't pay attention to me, he didn't want to be with me, I was a trophy to him. A prize," she spouted the therapy couch statements to paint a picture of her personal truth at that moment.

"Wasn't he working, didn't he invite you to the parties, the events? Did he not supply everything to you? The home, the lifestyle?" I said these things as they were shown to me. Stream of consciousness and talking out loud.

Two things were Grace's kryptonite. Her vanity and the truth.

She sat there, angry at me and the situation. She cried hard until she realized what it would do to her appearance. She sucked in her lips, looked up at the ceiling, and let out a deep, dramatic breath.

Her mother stepped forward. Evelyn appeared. She showed me how she passed. It was shown that there was chaos, screaming, and vanity. "I never should have thought I was worthy for a child," she said in such disdain as she turned her back on her daughter. "It would never be worth it," I heard the words of a woman angry, cold, and dismissive of the wonders of becoming a mother.

Healing symbols of Lilith in Sagittarius in the 8th house and Chiron in Pisces in the 12th house. One represents the power struggle of sexual health, expression, and relationship power dynamics, and the other indicates the loss of a parent early in life, past-life connection, and neglect. While both express deep loss and mistrust, they also diminish empathy and care.

I sat back and thought about how to present these very challenging aspects to her. The realization of several tough placements at the intersection of a breakthrough in her life. Knowledge like this is about understanding and empathy. Both of those things would be hard for her to recognize, let alone receive. She was sitting with someone who understood how she was as a person. The tough personality, the mistakes in relationships, burning down marriage to a wonderful man who accepted her who she was, mistakes and all. I took a deep breath and looked at her, keeping her composure.

"You're not broken," I said in a very monotone, non-judgmental statement.

She looked at me and winced her face. "Yes, I am. I broke my mother, I'm broke with no money, I'm bankrupt in my soul. The things I chased, the people I hurt. I could never be a mother, either. I lied to Jack. He just wanted to be a dad." Her voice trailed off as she ruined the rest of her makeup. The wails from a person understanding retribution decalcify your spine as you hear it. It makes you weak and nauseous. I offered her a water as I needed one for myself. Realizing she was in mourning and regret in equal measure. I gave her space. We sat in silence, drinking water, with only the occasional crinkle of the plastic bottles.

She looked at me with bloodshot eyes and cleared her throat, "Are all your readings like this?"

"No, but all of yours are," I said with a smile.

Grace blurted out a groggy laugh through her tears. "I don't know how to fix it other than break it," realizing her past performance in one statement. Somewhere in the space between what little we said, she realized it was what her mother did, too, in a way. I was searching for something to say. I wanted her grandmother to give me a word that gave her comfort. Maybe her mother connected with an apology, even wisdom. Nothing. I sat there as vulnerable as she had become.

"I was named after my grandfather, who died when my mother was five, and she never forgave me for it," I said in a monotone reality that I knew she would understand. To be a brave healer, you need to be vulnerable. To be vulnerable, you need to know your story and own it. I needed to show her what it looked like. In a sense, I acknowledged her ancestral wounds.

"How do you deal with it? How do I get past it all? I've been like this my whole life. Like I owe my mother praise and my grandmother respect. I hate my name!" she shouted through her gnashing teeth.

I realized why I spent time understanding astrology as well as my challenges. My own family 'stuff.' The guilt. The shame. The failures. There are no shortcuts, and the purpose of discovering how to use your gift can make you a powerful healer. Right now, I was sitting in the middle of Grace's breakthrough.

"The best day to plant a tree was twenty years ago. The next best day is today."

I let my words sit as she cleaned herself again. "I don't know what that means," she shrugged as she physically gave up in the moment.

"It means you can't go back and change anything, but you can make it look the way you want it to moving forward."

Vesta, the asteroid of learning, trine to Venus in Gemini in the third house. This brings a balance between one's inner devotion and external relationships, enhancing creativity, self-expression, and a sense of fulfillment and a radical acceptance of self-love.

I pulled my chair to be right in front of her. I took her hands in comfort. Asked her to take a deep breath. I asked her if she was ready.

"For what?" she snapped back.

"To continue to heal."

She looked at me as if I said the words she longed for her whole life. What she wanted was for someone to see her wounds. In reality, it was the first time she was willing to show them. I went to my computer and printed exactly what I needed. I walked into the bathroom and ripped the mirror off the wall. This worked for me and I hoped it would work for her. I walked into the room to her with her eyes closed. I handed her the sheet and sat down with the mirror on the floor.

"I want you to look in the mirror and say each one of those phrases and make eye contact."

"All of them?" she said as her voice broke. I nodded and held up the mirror in front of her. She drew from her acting classes and put herself into character. With bravery and even rebellion, she looked herself in the eye and began.

"I love you

I hear you

You didn't deserve this

I'm sorry

I forgive you

Thank you

You did your best"

The silence was deafening. I could see her mother and her grandmother again. Her mother was emotional, which is rare for spirit.

"I don't know what this is," she said to the paper. "All of these words are new to me, in this order." Grace was confused. Part because she was feeling her emotions. Part because she was vulnerable. But mostly, she realized she was able to do this on her own.

"Your mother is showing that she is proud of you." I honestly wasn't sure what it was she was showing, but knew she was watching.

Then I saw her grandmother say to her daughter, "Grace Evelyn, Grace."

I cleared my throat and delivered verbatim in tone and all, "Grace Evelyn, Grace."

She smiled at me and back at the mirror. "That is what my grandmother used to say all the time."

THE TOOL

The mirror exercise is a powerful tool to help break ancestral cycles, reinforce self-worth, and accept personal responsibility for healing and forgiveness.

1. Meditate and write down five phrases of impact that you need to hear. I love you, etc.

2. Shield yourself from the outside world and get in front of a mirror.

3. Say each phrase and look yourself in the eye as you say it. Repeat as often as you need. Start your day or end your day with it.

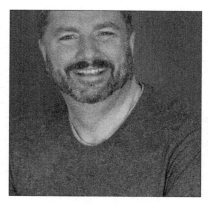

T Brandon Russ is a Certified Medium, but that's just the beginning. He is a Reiki Master Teacher, Certified Past Life Regressionist, and Certified Life and Spiritual Coach. Not to mention a Certified Sound Healer. He has taught over 200 different classes for Intuitive and Psychic Development. He has been a guest lecturer at mystical symposiums. As well as Ivy League colleges and universities. He has taught a college-accredited course about the Energy of Business. His first book, "Funny You Should Say That!" was well received as a raw and humorous confessional about becoming a Medium in modern times. His YouTube channel is filled with exploring Astrology, Tarot, and Socio-Economic energy on the state of the world. His live Message Circles across the country are entertaining, to say the least. Filled with uplifting connections and humor, you can tell how his greatest influence was Robin Williams. When he's not geeking out over his vinyl collection, a multitude of musical instruments, or writing new books or music, he's raising his three adopted sons.

To find out more about how he helps people on their path with readings, astrology and classes, his appearances, meditations, coaching programs, social media, and latest releases, visit www.tbrandonruss.com

CHAPTER 23

THE MAN IN THE STONE

CHIPPING AWAY TO FIND YOUR TRUE SELF

Joseph M. Fasi II, JD

"I look in the mirror through the eyes of the child that was me."

~ Judy Collins

MY STORY

"You're outstanding at what you do," said everyone. "You're loved so much!"

No way. They don't know me.

For years I'd heard these wonderful accolades that never resonated as truth. Then a dramatic event occurred seven years ago, and my life was shaken to the core—I hit rock bottom.

An addiction of mine finally came to the surface.

I already felt I had self-esteem issues, but I thought they were handled and not an issue. This day was the worst day of my life and the best day of my life. On that day, I began the journey that led to a true spiritual transformation and an introduction to what self-love means and how important it is to my life and relationships.

Flight attendants talk about putting your oxygen mask on before assisting another. The same is true for self-healing and wholeness. Self-care is not selfishness; it's critical to enable one to relate to others helpfully and honestly. In my opinion and experience, one cannot offer assistance to another without putting on your oxygen mask first.

I was told that this time of my life was when I needed to "Go big,"—to stop being dishonest with myself and take a closer look at my life. I was directed to when I was a child, and there, I found the answers to explain the hole in my heart that led to this time of my life.

I've always considered myself spiritually wise. After all, I had degrees in philosophy and theology. I was considered "religious" by the young people in my church and those I met in my daily life. They said I was an inspiration.

I must be fooling them again. I don't feel that way about myself. No way I am what they say I am.

In 1501, Michelangelo found and asked to carve a block of marble that had been discarded. The legend is that a young boy watched Michelangelo carve the block of marble for three years. When the now-famous sculpture of David was finished, the little boy asked, "Mister, how did you know there was a man inside that stone?"

That story intrigued me because it perfectly illustrates what was taking place within me over the past seven years. I thought I had it together and tried to appear confident and sure of myself. The fact is that I was not, and hence, I was uncomfortable when praised for being a fine man, a fine husband, a man of integrity, and a man who seemed to have it together. When I looked in a mirror, I knew the truth. In my heart, I was not any of these things. When told that I was loved, my first thought was always, *that's because you don't know me.*

The man I was to become, the man that was to evolve, was encased in a block of marble, figuratively speaking, of course, and work was needed to bring that man out.

"Go big" meant I let down my guard, asked for help, and was willing to face life honestly. I met with a therapist, found a life coach, and attended a men's meeting where I could be honest about my life and listen to how others overcame similar experiences and dilemmas and found the path to healing, wholeness, and joy.

I had to drop the façade of the intelligent and wise attorney and face the facts about the block of stone that contained the authentic, real me.

My therapist pointed out to me at one point that I thought I could get by in life with cunning and using my intellect. He asked me a question I'll never forget. "How has that worked out for you for the past 40 years?" Spot on observation.

He also asked, "What is the hole in your heart that you strive to fill so much?" That question stumped me. *What hole? What was I doing to fill that hole?*

A dear friend always told me I was enough. It sounded like some new-age babble to me. I didn't know what it meant. To make matters worse, I thought self-love was unattainable and not real anyway. And I didn't need self-love.

So, what was I to do? I needed to surrender and admit I needed help getting to know myself. I required a willingness to learn and grow. Thus, I began chipping away at the marble to find my true self.

As I was talking with my life coach and a group of men at our weekly meeting. A young man approached me and said, "I admire you so much, and I'd like to follow in your footsteps." My response was something to the effect of:

"You need to set your sights much higher, my friend."

My coach looked at me and asked why I'd say something like that. "Why would you not simply say thank you?" The truth was that I was uncomfortable because I didn't believe what he was saying about me.

The coach pointed out that whenever I made a mistake, I called myself *stupid* or "You're such an idiot."

"Joseph, you don't need anyone trying to put you down. You're doing a great job on your own."

He was correct. But why did I act this way? I needed to go way back and meet the much younger version of myself.

For most of my life, I had anger issues that manifested in different ways. I always attributed anger issues to my father's death when I was 12. As the oldest in the family, his death bothered me, but it didn't impact me until went to college.

But there had to be more.

I denied any trauma in my childhood. I idolized my dad. An immigrant to this country when he was a teen, he was a story of a self-made man fighting the prejudices immigrants faced in the 1920s. He couldn't do wrong in my eyes. After his death, I idolized him even more.

But it was time to face the facts.

To be as successful as he was meant, like many dads of the 1950s and 1960s, he was never home. He never played with me and never came to watch a ball game of mine. He was always working from 5 a.m. until late at night. Then he was gone. And I felt that I never measured up to his expectations.

The one person whose approval I sought would not be around to see me finally achieve something he talked about when I was little. He wouldn't see me graduate from college with honors, achieving a graduate degree or a law degree. That was his dream for me, and now it's a reality. But he wasn't there to see it. And I still felt I didn't have his approval. That was the hole in my heart I tried to fill, and I lived an angry life because I didn't know how. I was angry at myself for being such a perceived phony and incompetent person, pretending not to be these things and hating what I believed about myself.

As a child of immigrants in the 1950s, corporal punishment was the norm, and I experienced the same on many occasions. I recall being so incensed when I was spanked with a belt that I swore I'd deliver retribution when I grew up.

What occurred to me is that such actions, not just the punishments, led to my feeling I wasn't good enough. I believed I was a disappointment to my father. I was short, skinny, and not a good athlete. I cracked my front tooth when I was ten, and had a temporary crown that was yellow for seven years. I wore glasses and was the quintessential nerd in high school. School was not for me, and my grades were below average. I never had a date or got invited to a party, generally ate lunch by myself or with one other student in high school, and did not go to the senior prom.

Following eleventh grade, things changed. I grew three inches in height and gained fifty pounds of muscle. Tired of getting beat up, I joined the Boys' Club and learned how to box. Finally, something I was good at. For boys in the early 1970s, being well-built and a formidable boxer brought the respect I long sought. But it wasn't enough.

In college, things began to change. Students who didn't know me in my geeky nerd days liked and even admired me. I had dates with girls, and I was voted for president. The transformation began, and I was never seen as a nerd again. Except, I never saw myself in that way. I thought I was a terrific actor, fooling everyone. This feeling persisted throughout my adult life and into my fifties.

The real me was still in the stone. The real me was unknown to me, and the nerdy kid was all I had ever seen. When I looked in a mirror, I saw the unattractive, unathletic, unexceptional nerd. The difference was, I had him hidden away from the world (but not from myself).

It became clear to me that the little boy was still hurting and needed attention. The younger me needed reassurance that he was good enough and had value—that he was lovable.

How do I make this change?

How do I chip away at the stone and bring out my authentic, lovable self?

So, I began to catch myself calling myself stupid, dumb, and not very bright. None of which were true. It had to start there. I had to catch myself thinking these negative thoughts.

While physical fitness and appearance were paramount to me, I needed to focus on the spiritual part of me. That focus became first and foremost. I developed a spiritual transformation and gained conscious contact with God. I was a spiritual being having a human experience. Evolution was occurring, and it was healing and uplifting.

My routine of going to the gym at 5 a.m. was replaced with spending the first hour every day in quiet meditation and prayer. I learned about meditation and developing a focus on the spiritual side of my life. And I learned that being religious was of no value to me. What was of value was surrendering to God/Higher Power/The Universe, asking for help, and being open to receiving that help and those lessons.

Gradually, I began to learn to love who I am. I started to put the mask on my face first and felt the joy that comes from the peace of knowing I'm enough, from understanding what Carl Jung called "healing and wholeness," and embracing who I truly am, both the spiritual masculine and the spiritual feminine. The tool I used is explained in this chapter.

For the past few years, I've helped others uncover their journey, find the hole in their heart, chip away at the stone, find their authentic self-inside, and bring it to the pedestal of life, much like the statue of David in Florence.

Merely revealing your authentic self is a fraction of the journey. To genuinely love yourself involves embracing your true essence, having faith you're enough, welcoming love from others, and ultimately, extending that same love and acceptance to yourself like a big, warm embrace.

Once self-love became more than words, it anchored into who I am, not just what I say and do—it became real. Finally, I could stand in front of the mirror, look in my eyes, and say, "I love you" and "I'm proud of you" (and mean it). Life had joy, and I was loving it! I stopped dreading each day and eliminated the feeling of a dull life. The hole in my heart was full of life, love, acceptance, and deep understanding.

I want you to feel this same liberation, joy, and freedom, so I humbly provide this tool to free your authentic self from the stone.

THE TOOL

The tool I offer you, dear reader, is one I was taught, one that worked for me, and one that has helped others. It's simple and easy to use. It requires a willingness to try it and be open to its value.

The tool can be modified and used daily, and it will produce growth that you will feel and result in a life of joy and peace.

The tool is meant to help you meet your inner child. Find photos of yourself from when you were a child. I suggest making a photo album on your phone or a hard copy photo album. Include photos from when you were a baby, in first grade, high school, and even early college. It can even have pictures of you as a young adult. Then, while in your prayer or meditation time, look at those photos and talk to your younger self. Connect with the spirit of the young child that lives within you. Look at yourself with love and kindness—talk to that child.   Remember the pain felt as a child, confusion, fear, and anxiety, and tell your child that those days are gone. Give that child the respect and kindness that they deserve. Show your inner child the unconditional love you feel for them and promise they'll have your protection going forward.

When you look at yourself as a child, talk to yourself. Tell yourself,

"I have your back."

"You have nothing to be afraid of anymore."

"Look at how far we have come."

"No one will hurt you again. We are in this walk of life together."

"The best is yet to come."

It may seem difficult at first—trust in the process. Listen to what you may hear (or sense) being told by your inner child. Look at the photos, focus on them quietly, and spend time with yourself. Visualize yourself having a conversation with your inner child.

Close your eyes and see that child, look directly into the child's eyes, and feel the feelings again, but bring your adult self and life experiences into the conversation.

When I began to do this exercise, I felt awkward, but that feeling left me. I focused on the face and the eyes and remembered the pain and uncertainty. The face and emotions of my younger self came to life, and it was a spiritual conversation that was very real for me. It hit me that I wasn't ugly, I wasn't nerdy, I wasn't stupid, I wasn't a phony, I was capable, but for whatever reason, I did not feel it or believe it at that time. I began to feel peace and self-confidence in myself. I felt love for myself. I was finally being kind to myself. It helped me to journal my thoughts about what I felt and visualize my inner child.

The best *is* yet to come. I believe it for me and you. You'll have more growth, self-awareness, and respect than at any other time in your life. My message to you is that I'll emphasize how growth never stops. Thank God that growth and evolution never stops.

Suppose you're willing to make working the tool a priority for your life. It can be modified to whatever works and feels right for you. There is no one-size-fits-all when I'm talking about spiritual growth, development, and evolution.

There is so much more that I can offer you should you desire more in-depth guidance and coaching. It'd be my honor to work with you and witness your growth.

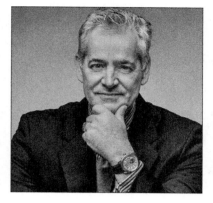

Joseph M. Fasi II is a practicing attorney who's been sharing his vision with others to assist the quest for a true spiritual transformation and a conscious connection with the spiritual part of oneself in the journey for healing and wholeness.

He holds a Bachelor of Arts in philosophy from Marquette University and a master's in religious education from Seattle University. He taught theology and philosophy in high schools for six years before obtaining his law degree from Stetson University College of Law. Joseph is a trial attorney handling trials throughout the country. In the past few years, he has worked with individuals who seek out his advice and guidance on many issues related to spiritual growth and personal development. He's described as an intuitive and spiritual individual with "emerging gifts."

This chapter is his first publication and certainly not his last.

When not sharing his gifts with others, he savors spending time with his daughters and grandchildren, riding his bicycle long distances, and traveling whenever possible.

To connect with Joseph and find out about how he helps one chip away at the stone and fine their true self, and receive a free gift go to:

Fasiwellness.com/hvw

CHAPTER 24

THE SECRET INGREDIENT IN THE KITCHEN: ENERGY

UNLOCK LIFELONG FOOD FREEDOM AND MAGNETIC VIBRANCY WITHOUT THE DIET

Hannah McKitrick

MY STORY

I teach people to create profound vibrance and freedom through cooking. Yet in September 2006, my body and mind were attacking themselves. I was diagnosed with Crohn's disease as I was getting ready to begin seventh grade. I had recently returned home from my first-ever sleep-away camp. I thought it'd be a week of play and connection. Instead, I was overcome with debilitating separation anxiety, trapped in my feelings, and suffocated from sadness. I couldn't cry hard enough. I remember going to the nurse to fake a sore throat, hoping it'd be my ticket home. When she put the thermometer underneath my tongue, I squeezed my tongue around it so tightly, willing the pressure to read as a fever. No luck!

As a child, I didn't have a say in the decision to stay at camp. I was stuck. I thought I'd feel better if I just made it home to my mom. Saturday couldn't come fast enough. After the longest week of my life, Saturday finally came. My parents picked me up—I made it home.

And then I noticed. The gut-wrenching sadness and anxiety were still there. I thought if I just made it home, I'd feel better. I soon learned that trauma doesn't pass through that easily.

The emotional pain became physical. I could hardly function—ridden with anxiety. It took over my life. I felt panicked going to school or anywhere else without my mom. My voice became hoarse for a whole year from crying so much. With all the social pressures to appear "normal," I had to ensure that approximately zero people aside from family knew what was happening internally.

I remember the distinct thoughts and feelings: *I can't scream hard enough* to *express the intensity of my sadness. My emotions don't make any sense. Why can't I escape the torture of my mind?*

It's no wonder that just weeks after returning home from sleep-away camp, my emotional pain manifested as a Crohn's diagnosis.

My body wouldn't absorb nutrients, and my mind only absorbed sadness. I disconnected from my body—disconnected from joy. I didn't know how to eat or how to be happy.

Fast forward seven years, and the doctors wanted to do surgery to remove part of my stomach. At this point, my life began shifting. I worked with a holistic practitioner to use food to heal my gut. I had minimal hope going into this "too good to be true" promise of a healthy gut void of hospitalizations and surgery.

I followed the rigid food regime prescribed. For months, I consumed only certain cooked vegetables, whole grains, and water.

I again felt trapped.

My body was finally receiving the healing nutrients it needed. However, my mind and soul were stripped dry from joy. **I realized how much of my daily excitement revolved around food.**

Nothing felt as fun anymore—hanging with friends, going out to eat, traveling, and parties all felt lackluster. I felt like I was making a scene by always packing "special" food for celebratory events. Not only did I feel segregated, but being surrounded by the temptation of foods like pizza, crab cakes, or truffle cheese felt torturous!

It was paradoxical. I was finally able to reconnect to my body. I was eating a "picture-perfect" healthy diet but still suffering. The restriction of that diet cut me off from what my mind and soul deeply desired. I didn't feel good. I didn't feel healthy.

I didn't want to choose between being healthy or enjoying my life.

I didn't want to choose between a healthy gut or going out to dinner with my friends.

I wanted to feel good in my body *and* feel happy!

I didn't know if I could have both.

The doctors definitely didn't think so.

But I sure as hell was going to try! My sanity was worth that much.

I took what I learned from the gut-healing diet and distilled it to "vegetables and whole foods" as my baseline eating routine. It sounds so simple, so elementary. But health and nutrition can appear complicated. I spent years prior overanalyzing what to eat and juggling conflicting opinions. Simplifying nutrition into these two categories allowed me to stop overthinking which foods would give my body vibrancy. Instead, when choosing to eat well, I could pull out my nutrition cheat sheet (vegetables and whole foods) to satisfy that need.

This newfound knowledge gave me simple access to vibrancy without the drama.

I intuitively front-loaded my routine with these foods to give my body what it needed. This routine allowed space for my joy-led intuition to guide other food choices solely to satiate my mind and soul's desires.

This flexibility wasn't what the doctor ordered. But it changed my life and gave me freedom.

I wasn't bypassing my body's needs. I had learned to incorporate them with flexibility to remove the drama. There was no rigidity.

I was able to bring back food flexibility with what my emotions desired. This looked like a morning run followed by a green protein smoothie with some peanut butter-stuffed pretzels. Or a veggie-heavy dinner followed by a homemade cookie. This is what my body wanted to eat (vegetables and fruit), balanced with what my mind craved (crunchy pretzels) and what my soul was yearning for (a warm cookie).

This is food freedom. This is my intuitive health. This embodied balance shifted my energy. This daily energy shift continues to sustain my healing. It's been 12 years since I've had a flare-up.

I felt like I finally cracked the code where I could have it all: joy, freedom, flavor, vitality, and comfort.

Out of my desire to "have it all," my specialty became bringing gourmet flavor to vegetables and whole foods to optimize mind, body, and soul health. I chose foods with higher vibrations (plants and whole foods). I also chose foods that permitted freedom of convenience and cravings (pizza, extra cheese, Prosecco, etc.)

I enhanced every food I could and got creative with my meals. I savored the flavors of smokey cauliflower tacos adorned with sautéed caramelized onions and black beans, crowned with a luscious avocado crèma. I delighted in the comfort of roasted eggplant stacks layered with farro, creamy goat cheese, and vibrant pistachio arugula pesto. I indulged in the zesty lemon pesto spaghetti squash accompanied by artichoke hearts, sun-dried tomatoes, crispy chickpeas, and more than a healthy "pinch" of Parmesan cheese for creamy decadence.

I luxuriated in being able to create these types of mouth-watering dishes that also left me feeling light. The flavor, the creativity, and the deliciousness brought me so much joy. I infused joy into the ingredients, the cooking process, and the food.

And my body noticed.

For years, my inflammation markers were elevated past the normal range. Out of curiosity, I recently looked at a graph of my inflammation labs with data spanning 18 years. I noticed two things. Improvement in my labs began when I incorporated my intuitive health routine. But remission began precisely once I added cooking to my mix. I was in awe at the correlation.

The intuitive health routine of flexibility, flavor, and simplicity was a great starting point for reducing inflammation. It allowed my health to feel easy.

But cooking embedded this shift on a deeper level, sustaining my labs at an all-time low.

Cooking became the easiest path toward mind, body, and soul alignment, where I got to feel fit in my body and vibrant in my mind without deprivation.

In the kitchen, the sizzle on the pan and the fragrant symphony of spices transcended my overthinking mind and brought me into my body. With each chop of the knife and swirl of the spoon, I embarked on a journey of pleasure, where nourishing my body became a sacred ritual.

Cooking with high-vibrational foods (plants, whole foods) helped me feel grounded and light as I became infused with the very essence of these ingredients. It permeates my being.

It'll do that for you, too, and more.

Cooking with flavor increases your pleasure and enjoyment and gets you excited about food.

The act of cooking with your hands gets you out of the racing mind and into the body.

The creativity and sensory stimulation bring you into the present moment and your true self.

Cooking creates a major energy shift, and digesting that food magnifies it.

Food is an energy amplifier traveling through the system and magnetizing out the aura. It affects everything and everyone around you.

The humble meal works in the background to carry the energy it was prepared with, to carry not only nutrients but also love. That love gets absorbed inwards and emulated out. It's alchemy.

And it worked.

I felt aligned; I felt connected, and I was a clear vessel.

It allowed me to digest the joy on a deeper level.

From depressed to exuberant. From hospitals to complete health.

It creates an embodied shift.

Cooking food is powerful. Food affects the emotional, physical, and energetic state. Moreover, your emotional and energetic state also affects your food.

I spent so much of my adolescence feeling anxious and sick that it's now crucial for me to have an outlet that infuses so much joy into my mind, body, and soul. Being playful in the kitchen saved my life in more ways than one.

It shifted my state into joy and vibrancy in a way therapy, meditation, or tears never could. I don't eat perfectly, and I don't have to. The frequency I emulated around food permitted all foods of my choosing to be healing.

The joy and intention I bring to food carry an energetic signature surpassing labels and rules. I'm no longer trapped.

This is part of the power and magic I help others create around food in my business, My Intuitive Health. I found such freedom in this new way of eating, in this new way of being, that I needed to share it with others. I wanted to create an experience for others where they could step out of any "heavy" thoughts around life and food and into pure light-heartedness. So they could also make health accessible, effortless, and fun. So they could have more alignment and be a grounding rod of light. Cooking is my favorite way to create this shift.

Food is my main instrument to help not only myself carry and sustain joy, but to help others emulate the frequency of light.

Food continues to be the vessel that has the power to heal all parts of us: emotionally, physically, and spiritually. And I, in turn, continue to be the vessel that energetically heals all foods.

It's a partnership.

It's a dance.

Food is so strongly linked to emotion.

Cooking is linked to shifting your state of being.

It's the perfect formula for a mind-body shift.

THE TOOL

Use this framework and reflection questions to create your intuitive health blueprint to shift your energy to vibrancy, joy, groundedness, and freedom. Then embed it into your body through cooking!

1. SIMPLE NUTRITION:

Simple nutrition will shift your energy into vibrancy.

I define simple nutrition as vegetables and whole foods (one-word ingredients) like nuts, seeds, legumes, fruits, and whole grains. These foods are the most gut-healing. They are closest to the earth and contain the highest amounts of frequency. Their vibrations are higher than processed boxed foods. Digesting high-frequency foods gets your body ready to hold your next up-level. This food grounds you more deeply.

I simplified nutrition into two categories because complications lead to being overwhelmed, which increases cortisol and slows digestion. Simplifying nutrition will replace the mental mind chatter with ease and clarity to knowing how to eat in a way that supports your body. Of course, every person is different—permission to trust your body's reactions to food.

JOURNAL PROMPTS:

- *How do I feel physically when eating vegetables and whole foods?*
- *How would my life change if I didn't have to overanalyze how to eat well and just focus on these two categories?*
- *What foods do I enjoy that fall into the simple nutrition category of vegetables and whole foods?*

2. FLAVOR:

Flavor will shift your energy into joy and happiness.

Flavor is crucial to your emotional satisfaction. Your emotional satisfaction is crucial to your health. When you eat something flavorful, you exude the emotions of bliss, excitement, and happiness. When something is flavorful, these associated emotions radiate out of your being. Also, bringing flavor into simple nutrition helps make eating well intuitive and crave-worthy. You'll no longer need to *force* yourself to eat well. Instead, you'll *want* to because it's so delicious!

My biggest tip for flavor: homemade sauces on vegetables, salads, or grain bowls! BONUS: I've included my favorite lemon basil pesto recipe below—try it out!

3. ROUTINE:

A routine will shift your energy into calmness and groundedness.

Now you have your little mental cheat sheet that can quickly guide you to "What will add health to my body?" With this, you can form a food routine that makes you feel good physically. You can lean on your base of empowerment whenever you want to feel physically your best.

A healthy eating routine gives you the freedom to enjoy other foods you crave, knowing that the foundation will be waiting for you. It allows a greater freedom of choice without negative effects.

It's not a diet that you have to follow. It's a way of life where you feel empowered whenever you want. Creating a routine allows this structure to hold your health. Your mind will no longer need to overanalyze what to eat. No mind chatter, no debating, just knowing that this foundation of health is there for you when you need to feel good in your body.

JOURNAL PROMPT:

- Create a hypothetical outline of foods that make you feel empowered. Start with one day or even one meal. It could be a healthy salad for lunch filled with chickpeas, artichokes, feta, peppers, and roasted sweet potatoes, or it could be a green smoothie for breakfast or a healing chicken soup for dinner. What makes you feel best? These foods will be your routine to create your feel-good health that you can weave into your day.

4. FLEXIBILITY:

Flexibility will shift your energy into fun and freedom.

"Health is a state of complete physical, mental, and social well-being, not merely the absence of disease or infirmity. The enjoyment of the highest attainable standard of health is one of the fundamental rights of every human being without distinction of race, religion, political belief, economic or social condition." ~World Health Organization.

We can't systematize eating—we're not meant to, and it won't be effective if we try.

Bringing flexibility to a simple health structure will shift your frequency to freedom and fun. It creates a sustainable approach to health. Incorporating flexibility allows you to live fully and presently without bracing for the impact of foods, treats, or events you "should" avoid. Intentionally incorporating flexibility removes any guilt or shame that may linger around what's "healthy." Often, letting yourself eat foods for nostalgia, convenience, or desire is the healthiest thing you can do for yourself. It's being authentic to your mind and soul.

JOURNAL PROMPT:

- *What would allow you more freedom with your healthy eating routine? Define some food rituals that feel important and fun for you, regardless of their physical health benefits. Is it dessert? Friday night pizza?* Remember, it's not your standard for eating every meal. It's your wiggle room that you're outlining so that you can consciously enjoy while being backed by your routine above. Becoming aware of these will allow you to mindfully and peacefully indulge in a less restrictive way.

5. EMBODIMENT:

Cooking will embody vibrancy, joy, happiness, groundedness, calmness, freedom, and fun into your being.

This is arguably the most important step! Right now, you're reading and absorbing information through your mind. Following the above guidelines helps to create more happiness, pleasure, and food freedom. The next step is to embed vibrancy into your frequency to sustain intuitive health. This is done through cooking. The embodied process of cooking in this way, with your hands, and digesting that food will sustain this shift on a cellular level.

Action item: try out this recipe and notice how you feel!

HARVEST SALAD WITH ROASTED SQUASH AND FARRO TOSSED IN LEMON PESTO

INGREDIENTS:

3 cups of arugula

1 delicata squash, sliced into ¼ inch half-moons

1 tablespoon olive oil

½ teaspoon garlic powder

½ teaspoon dried rosemary

3 ounce crumbled goat cheese

1 avocado, cubed

Salt and pepper, to taste

For the Farro:

1 cup of dried farro

2.5 cups of vegetable broth

Salt and pepper, to taste

For the Pesto:

1 cup, fresh basil, packed

2 cloves of garlic

Juice of 1 lemon

1-2 teaspoons of honey

⅓ nuts (walnuts, pine nuts, cashews, pistachios etc.)

⅓ cup olive oil

Salt and pepper, to taste

INSTRUCTIONS:

For the Squash:

Preheat the oven to 425 degrees. Line one sheet tray with parchment paper. Add the sliced squash and season with oil, salt, pepper, garlic powder, and rosemary. Roast for 15-20 minutes, then flip and roast for another 15-20 minutes until tender and beginning to brown and char.

For the Farro:

Add 1 cup of farro with 2 1/2 cups of broth to a pot over high heat. Bring to a boil and then reduce to a simmer. Cook for about 15 minutes or until the liquid has just been absorbed. Season the farro with salt, pepper, and a tablespoon of the pesto.

For the Pesto:

In a food processor, combine all the ingredients for the pesto sauce and pulse until smooth. Taste for seasoning and adjust (salt, pepper, honey). If the mixture is too thick, you can add more oil.

To assemble:

Layer arugula, farro, squash, goat cheese, sliced avocado, and any extra nuts you have. Toss with lemon basil pesto and enjoy!

For more recipes, download my favorite 15-minute recipes:

https://myintuitivehealth.com/15-minute-recipes-sign-up/

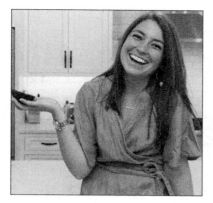

Hannah McKitrick is a "Kitchen Psychic" who's paving a new way of health that ditches the diet and instead combines energy with food to bring more lightness into the entire being: physically, emotionally, and spiritually. She's trained in energy work and intuition development, studied Eastern medicine at the Academy of Healing Nutrition, went to culinary school in Italy, and healed her gut of Crohn's disease through food.

Her business, My Intuitive Health, has helped people worldwide nourish their "soul health" from the inside out, using food and connection as the catalyst that raises their vibration. She holds a healing yet playful space for others to have a ridiculous amount of fun while cooking healthy meals during her transformational cooking programs and culinary wellness retreats in southern Italy. Hannah has lived through some heavy seasons in life, so she's now obsessed with creating experiences that help others *feel and be* lighter. Life isn't nearly as serious as the mind makes it out to be! What if the healthiest thing you could do was go to Italy and eat some pasta?

Connect with Hannah:

Website: https://myintuitivehealth.com/

Instagram: https://www.instagram.com/hannah.mckitrick/

Facebook: https://www.facebook.com/hannah.mckitrick/

LinkedIn:

https://www.linkedin.com/in/hannah-mckitrick-91649573/

CHAPTER 25

FIND YOUR BALANCE

A COLORFUL RECIPE FOR YOUR SOUL

Tammy "TLC" Lynn Calderon,
Color Master, Universal Angel Channeler

*The Universe orchestrates itself to
accommodate your "colorful" picture of reality!*

MY STORY

Before my spiritual awakening as TLC, the heart and channeler of the universal color language, I was a young mother running a successful home daycare with my three boys and five other little ones. I offered preschool and a music class, and a tumble gym bus came once a week. Until the day a windblown Jacuzzi cover slammed me over the head, aggravating a pre-existing neck injury and turning my life into a train wreck.

Previous major scoliosis and neck surgeries had reinforced the belief doctors had all the answers, and this time was no different. I had a strong feeling that there was something wrong with my neck. The doctors started treating me for anxiety, not my neck, which led them to prescribe pills for me.

Why are they not listening to me? It's my neck!

Against my intuition, I listened to the doctors. After a horrendous year on a mixture of prescription medications, I was unable to function in any capacity due to a chemical imbalance caused by poly-pharmacy.

My mind was a train wreck, and my body craved balance. I didn't feel loved or supported, and I wasn't speaking my truth. Later, the angels shared their wisdom: *Everyone loves you; they're just not aware of it yet.* The truth was, neither was I. One night, I surrendered and asked God to take the pain away—or else, I was ready to let go if that was the way of it.

A voice as loud as a freight train screeched inside my head:

If you take another pill, it will kill you!

The thundering voice demanded my attention with such intensity that fear engulfed my entire being, stopping me in my tracks. *Who is this voice? Can I trust it?* It seemed to know a more profound truth. Now peaceful and calm, the voice offered me a choice: *Choose love or fear: If you choose love, we'll lead you to be an angel on Earth.*

The tone of reassuring authority—as if it knew me better than I knew myself—made me feel safe and loved. When I tuned into that voice - my soul, I felt a knowing that I could trust it.

At that moment, over 20 years ago, I chose to quit the pills cold turkey. My story isn't about pills, though they were part of the drama, the great pain I created to awaken into the truth of who I am: unconditional divine love. Trusting that voice guided me to the invisible healing energy of colors and crystals connected to a universal intelligence that always supports me and feeds my soul—where this story begins.

I felt empty, unable to function. I didn't recognize myself, a stranger to my reflection. I only knew that I was a mother with three boys and had responsibilities. I needed my life back. Left in the dark of a confusing withdrawal, I turned to the persistent voice. I asked: *How can I escape this overwhelming fear and unbearable pain?*

The voice spoke softly: *Create a new reality within this space—an angel story.*

I emerged as TLC, my initials, but also my new identity. The angels promised to reveal answers and solutions, enabling me to act from a place of love in every experience. Through their guidance, I learned to love myself and became a mirror of love, seeing everyone's light and innocence. Love is the sole path to harnessing your power. When you don't choose love, you unwittingly surrender your power.

From the dark night of the soul, I deliberately claimed, "I choose love!" Committing to love, I felt a power surge unlike anything I'd ever experienced.

Whenever I felt stuck, it was my signal to go inward and ask: *Angels, show me what I'm not seeing.*

Trust flowed like a gentle river, guiding me into a new landscape of angelic simplicity. Stepping into the beautiful rainbow realm of the angels, I found comfort, belonging, and hope. I saw the promise of a world filled with colors, a world I yearned to live in.

Is this Heaven on Earth? Why wait for Heaven? I can create it on Earth!

I tuned into the voice and heard: *Go to Florida; you'll transform there.*

Though scared, I trusted the angels, believing they'd guide me to healing and transformation for myself and my sons. Sure enough, my whole heart opened up in Sarasota, Florida, and all my pain and old energy started leaving my body. I spent the next two years healing and balancing with *Qigong*, Rolfing, Reiki, and massage therapy to get to the truth:

I am whole and complete

I know what to do

One of my healers continuously emphasized that I was filled with spiritual energy and encouraged me to trust and allow it to flow through me. I wondered what she was seeing that I didn't see. Every healer I was led to showed me a forgotten piece of myself. *Is transformation remembering who you are?*

Immersing myself in The Work of Byron Katie, I deeply connected with her teachings. During one of her talks, she referred to the awakening inside of her as "It." I was so moved that I couldn't resist running to the stage. Breathless, I exclaimed, "You knew that 'It' woke up inside me." She replied, "It was obvious." *Who is the It? Is It the voice? What is she seeing?* Still, It was a huge confirmation of my awakening experience.

During an airline flight, I read a book titled *Why Am I Afraid to Tell You Who I Am?* The revelation flashed before me in an airport mirror, and I burst into laughter—finally seeing myself without any of the self-imposed filters; the mask was gone. "I see you and your beauty," I said as I looked in the mirror.

In a dream during a stay at a hotel in Asheville, North Carolina, I dreamt of an empty hole inside of me. I was filling this void with all my negative experiences and emotions, collecting them, and feeling burdened by their weight. Then, there was a shift. Instead, I began filling this space with the colorful, angelic energy of joy, beauty, power, and love. I began to feel lighter and freer.

Upon waking, I shared this insight with a friend, tears streaming down my face. I realized I was the monster in the closet. I fostered fear within myself, and it became vividly clear in this dream that I had to choose fear or love. I filled myself up with love and was liberated from fear and suffering.

I whispered: *Thank you, angels. Keep showing me how to love myself; I am willing to learn. I am my soulmate. I am the one that I have been searching for.*

The angels revealed that colors hold purpose, intentions, and unique strengths within us. It felt like a divine download from the angelic realm, filling me with vibrational color information. I felt a growing curiosity about each color. I began intentionally feeding myself with colors giving me access to the Universal One Field - a world I had never known before. The Voice of knowing was divinely informing me of a higher energy solution and pathway for my life. My relationship with color became my life's passion. Feeling colors raise my vibration, and trusting my soul's resonance became my new way of life.

Angels, show me how to have this energy around me all the time!

That year, at the Tucson Gem Show, my angels guided me to a rough-handed bearded Arkansas miner. He showed me how to embed quartz crystals into a colorful plant-based resin.

Not just any crystals–Atlantean crystals, which seem to have unique energy to balance chakras. Quartz holds color frequencies and information and amplifies these frequencies into your field, raising your vibration.

Aha, this is it! I can wear the pendant and have color frequencies, crystals, and angels around me all the time.

This is when I birthed my Quantum Balance Crystal pendants. I program my QBCs with specific healing frequencies, including the Schumann resonance (grounding to Earth's frequency) and the love vibration (528 Hz), which quantum leaps your energy into balance.

A healer pointed out that I wasn't grounded. *What's grounding?* Deeply connected spiritually—strongly resonating with purple and magenta—I often struggled to inhabit my physical body. The angel color download said red is for grounding: the root energy center. *Let's see if it works.* I wore a red pendant, imagining myself as a tree with red roots extending from the soles of my feet, connecting me to the earth. I began to understand color as a tool of interconnectedness in this vast universe of energy. *The universe supports me!* I am willing to embrace change, open up to new possibilities, focus on a sustainable foundation of love, and always respond—not react—to the world.

Working at a health food store, I wore red for a month and felt "nudges" about which customers to connect with. I declared, "Red is my money magnet!" To my amazement, I sold 12 pendants to a single customer! I felt successful and fully present in the manifestation of red energy.

I continued wearing red, and to my surprise, my oldest son joined me on this journey. He designed my logo, brochure, and website. Within the year, the pendants reached 24 countries. "Balance your energy" became the mantra, connecting with others through the simple invitation: "Let me show you."

Red works! Prosperity is everywhere.

Steve, a lanky, good-looking guy, walked quickly through the exhibitor room on his way to David Avocado Wolfe's presentation in 2009. As if yanked back by an invisible cord, he halted abruptly in front of my Quantum Balance Crystals display of 12 colored pendants with unbridled curiosity.

"What's going on here?"

"I feel a buzz around this booth! There was color! TLC (in tie-dye, of course) was doing this *thing* with people. The energy just drew me in!" he recalls.

The buzz Steve felt was in resonance with my colorful QBCs.

"We're doing balance tests. These pendants balance your energy. Let me show you."

"I don't know what a balance test is," Steve admitted. "But I'm a roofer—I'm interested in balance!"

I explained, "The balance test is a kinesiology tool I use to feel and connect with your energy. Pressing down on your hand while you stand as sturdy as a tree, your equilibrium either feels weak or strong. When I surge with your energy, a color flows through me; the one that your divine intelligence shows me will balance your energy into a structured, coherent state."

"Without a crystal in my hand, I was teeter-tottering," Steve continues. "I didn't realize how unbalanced I was! Then TLC put the aqua higher heart QBC pendant in my hand—boom! Without any effort, not trying to be macho or strong, my equilibrium was instantaneously stabilized. I was in an easy sustainable energy field of immovable balance. My mind was blown. I *felt* the quantum field and its effect! I'd been curious about this infinite, invisible energy for some time. Now, I'm having this amazing experience with "TLC.""

Aqua Works!

Higher Heart Intelligence guides me.

What Steve didn't know at our first encounter was that I'd been wearing an 'Orange' QBC pendant for the past month to attract my soulmate! The angels told me I had to clear old relationship patterns so I wouldn't manifest my ex again. I asked the angels "to show me a man who knew I was coming from my heart." I'd felt an enormous shift and trusted that I would soon attract a healthy relationship. Steve showed up just seven days later—from 'Orange' County, California! Steve felt my heart and said: "TLC knows," and I knew he was the one.

Orange works!

Trust the Process

Fifteen years ago, Steve walked into my booth and never left. My life partner designed the 12-color tulle roof of my rainbow booth, a true masterpiece of the angelic playground within! The rainbow booth has allowed me to fully live my purpose and embrace my new energy life with the Angels. I have expanded in many ways and now share my color angel downloads with my world family under the rainbow in my booth. "Look for us under the rainbow!" we always say.

My Angel Board of Directors and I co-created QBCs from the invisible quantum energy field surrounding us. They showed me the 12 Color-rich Tools for Awakening, each carrying universal energy and frequencies. Wearing them lets you feel a deeper presence resonating within your energy centers.

It was time to share my message about the transformative power of color with a larger audience. Still, the mere thought of uttering my name in front of others sent waves of fear coursing through me. In one of the first self-development workshops I attended, I had to say, "I am courageous," in front of the class, triggering an instinctual urge to flee.

I finally stopped arguing with my soul's inner voice, and I said: *yes, I will bust through my biggest fear.* I then enrolled to be a speaker at the Conscious Life Expo in Los Angeles, *the* major metaphysical show!

OMG. . .Angels, show me what I am not seeing; show me I am a speaker!

They have a sense of humor!

Just wing it, you know what to do;

It's inside of you.

So, for the month prior, I wore yellow, blue, and black pendants strung together into a trinity necklace —yellow symbolizing courage: "I can, I am enough, I am a master and leader of self." Blue is communication, stillness, and peace, "I speak my truth." Black signifies healthy boundaries and bolsters my energy field, warding off outside influences. My presentation was a smashing success, and many came back to my colorful rainbow booth. I felt the terror of public speaking leave my body. I was free and now on a journey to bust through all my fears using my yellow power within.

Yellow, blue, and black works!

I am unstoppable!

At my booth or online, I interact with people and feel their energies. I tune in connecting to your divine presence and a color surges throughout my field. I've learned to trust the first color I see and feel. I may be guided to a recipe of colors that your soul sees as its best ingredients in moving you forward. I am always delighted at the amazed responses when I feel the color that you already know. I was simply the channel and your confirmation. *We are connected!*

I am here as an angel on Earth, a color master and channeler, to remind—myself first and then you—to use the consciousness and energy of color as a divine tool. Why? So that you may target and create an intentional lifestyle of beauty for yourself that is aligned with your soul's fulfillment.

It's all energy! Let's go!

We never miss our target!

While this story I've shared is uniquely mine, you may feel these words and insights resonating within you on a deeper level because they came through the angelic realm.

We are all angels in the playground of color. I'm deeply grateful for our connection and time together!

THE TOOL

COLORS FOR AWAKENING

Find a quiet and comfortable space to connect with the color that resonates with your manifestation journey. Close your eyes and center yourself with deep, relaxing breaths.

Feel the subtle vibrations of the color calling out to you, recognizing its alignment with your unique energy signature. Allow yourself to receive the color, sensing a connection.

Set your intention to attune to the color that'll support and empower you on your path of manifestation. Trust in the universe to guide you to the perfect match that resonates deeply with your soul's journey.

Let's begin:

1. **Centering:** Feel yourself fully supported as you take a good slow deep breath in. Receiving the breath into the body and allowing it to circulate and be. Let your breath breathe you.

2. **Invoking Presence:** Invite your spiritual guides, angels, and ascended masters to join you. Feel their loving presence surrounding and enveloping you in their divine energy.

3. **Heart Center Activation:** Now, shift your focus to your heart center, the sacred space within you where your true essence resides. This is home, your sanctuary of love and compassion.

4. **Connecting with Your Color:** With your attention anchored in your heart, ask your guides to reveal a color that resonates with your soul's journey.

5. **Visualizing the Color:** As the color emerges, feel its presence surrounding and energizing you with vibrant vitality. Visualize this color filling your entire being, illuminating every cell and fiber. Let it infuse you with its unique qualities and vibrations.

6. **Acknowledging Sacred Connection:** This color is a sacred gift from the angelic realm, symbolizing your divine connection and purpose. Treasure it deeply and allow it to guide you on your path.

7. **Wearing the Color:** If you have a quantum balance pendant or any object representing your chosen color, hold it close to your heart. Feel its resonance amplifying the connection between you and the angelic realm, anchoring you into the New Earth energies.

8. **Gratitude and Closure:** Take a moment to express gratitude to your guides for their presence and guidance throughout this meditation. You can return to this space anytime you seek clarity, comfort, or connection.

9. **Slowly return:** When ready, gently bring your awareness back to the present moment. Wiggle your fingers and toes. Take a good deep breath. Slowly opening your eyes, feeling refreshed, renewed, and deeply connected to your color.

Thank you for joining me on this colorful journey.

If you're curious to explore further, I invite you to visit my website at qbcrystals.com to discover all 12 universal color frequencies and delve into the rich language of color!

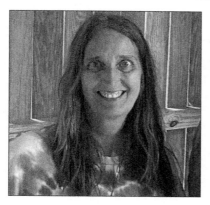

Tammy "TLC" Lynn Calderon, As the visionary founder of Quantum Balance Crystals, I'm affectionately known as TLC, the Heart of QBC. Growing up on a pig farm in South Dakota, I developed a deep connection with nature and animals. With my dad raising 1,000 pigs annually and living in a small town with just 350 people, we certainly had more pigs than people! At age 7, I had my first horse and learned the importance of fearlessness and connection with animals. After earning a commercial economics degree from South Dakota State University, I was selected as one of twelve for the Walt Disney World College Program, where I absorbed Walt Disney's guest relations principles.

My passion for color and its healing potential led me to establish Quantum Balance Crystals. Through energetic pendants, I strive to bring forth angelic vibrations and create a world that's magical, inspiring, and colorful—a "Wonderful World of Color." My mission is to use color to enhance well-being and connect individuals to their hearts and the universal energy field, empowering them to share this connection with others.

As a Color Reiki Master and advanced color medicine practitioner, I have mastered my skills in energy healing and understand the intentional impact color can have on our lives.

I offer free virtual color readings to align you with the universal flow, helping you connect with yourself and share that connection with your friends and family. Whether through virtual sessions or in-person conferences and expos, I am available as a speaker to share this transformative color information with you and your groups.

Join me on this colorful journey:

Website: qbcrystals.com/hvw

Phone: +1 (702) 499 7067

Email: qbcplanet@gmail.com

Instagram: qb_crystals

View my socials, meditations, and testimonials on Linktree: linktr.ee/qbcrystals

I offer free color readings; you may book a session on my website or via phone!

Feel It to Believe It

CLOSING CHAPTER

NOURISHING YOUR BODY TEMPLE

Lainie Sevante Wulkan

"Nourishing yourself in a way that helps you blossom
in the direction you want to go is attainable,
and you are worth the effort."

~ Deborah Day

Compelling, traumatic, awakening, transformative, and enlightening—
these are the words and more of the stories just shared in *High Vibrational
Wellness—Intuitive Healing Therapies to Nourish Your Body Temple*.

To move toward the next phase of one's healing journey, it takes a
true spiritual warrior's willingness to be honest with oneself. When you
can look at your wounds and recognize the meaning and messages of
their existence, then the road to understanding yourselves as sovereign
beings becomes easier to navigate.

The authors shared wide-open vulnerability, which felt both gut-
wrenching and challenging to read and other times deeply heartwarming
and inspiring. Each had a different personal story to bring you to the
same conclusion: Change begins inside and healing is found in the least
unlikely of circumstances.

When we can quiet our minds and begin the process of activating our
intuition, the sacred dialogue within our divine selves, we become better
equipped to activate the next steps of healing in our multiple bodies—
emotional, mental, physical, and spiritual.

EMPS wellness is the totality of all four bodies working together in one accord. It's the sound of a perfect symphony where the instruments are working together to create a perfect rhythm. It's the centered alignment of all forces working in unison for the highest good of all concerned. It's knowing that you're nourishing your body temple with the highest of respect, honor, and reverence that a Divine being would do when greater awareness is present. This is what we sought to provide—a moment of presence to awaken your mind, body, and spirit to the greater truths that await you when you are ready to say yes! Yes, to more love for yourself, yes to greater connection to the Divine, and yes to the knowing that all you ever needed is already inside. When the student is ready, the teacher will appear.

Food, in all its facets, was a teacher and took on many meanings in these chapters. Our intuitive food therapists, health coaches, and chefs taught you the importance of high vibrational wellness with what's consumed literally in your mouth. Our multi-modality healers, which included Reiki masters, nurses, essential oil specialists, mediums, shamans, Yoga teachers, energy healers, hypnotherapists, astrologers, numerologists, life coaches, and more, taught you how to metaphorically feed your mind and how you feed your soul is also essential to nourishing the body temple.

Consider the tools offered by the authors as multiple recipes for self-love. When practiced regularly, these nutritious and delicious healing options will lead you home to the kitchen of your heart for infinite high vibrational wellness. Thank you.

"Your relationship with love is your relationship with the essence of who you are. It affects your relationship with your body and your relationship with food. When you realize that you are a spirit and that this body is a temple, then you want to treat it well."

~ Marianne Williamson

Blessings of gratitude to each of you who embarked on this high-vibrational sojourn into wellness. We're grateful and blessed to be part of your journey. May your next chapter in intuitive wellness be healthy, joyful, and bright. And so it is…

AUTHOR RESOURCES

I welcome you to visit:
https://CenterforIntuitiveFoodTherapy.com/HVW
for a listing of our authors' contact information
and a video/audio welcome message.

INFINITE GRATITUDE

As a sovereign community of like-minded beings, we can move mountains. It's more than "when two or more are gathered, we are strong." It's the willingness to hear the call of resonance and attract to its field.

This happened when 25 authors from across the globe said yes to *High Vibrational Wellness – Intuitive Healing Therapies to Nourish Your Body Temple*. It does "take a village" to create, produce, and manifest a project such as HVW into form and bring it emotionally, mentally, physically, and spiritually into being. Kudos to all who have come together for this divine appointment.

Gratitude goes beyond measure. Everyone brought their strengths and vulnerabilities to showcase their chapter to the world. Authors brought their gifts of healing, drawing from their areas of weakness, traumas, learning, and growth. For this and more, I thank you.

I am deeply grateful for this collaboration, and my absolute honor to have more opportunities together to share our works for humanity in the future.

With deep love and appreciation,

Lainie Sevante Wulkan

THE WORKS OF LAINIE SEVANTE WULKAN

As a multi–modality healer, Sevante offers private sessions both in person and online in the areas of:

- Oracle Readings
- Food Healing
- Advanced Theta Healing
- Law of Attraction
- EFT/Tapping
- Life Coaching
- Spiritual Counseling
- Enlightened Business Consulting
- Customized Recorded Meditation Sessions

BOOKS, MEDITATIONS & PUBLICATIONS

- The Food Healing Oracle Deck®, Vol I (available in hard copy at CIFTofficial.com)
- SECOND HELPINGS—The Food Healing Oracle Deck®, Vol II (available in hard copy at CIFTofficial.com)
- Smoothies – Nourishing Wisdom Beyond the Blend (available in hardcopy or digital at CIFTofficial.com or Amazon.com)
- Top Exotic Foods for Natural Healing–Power-Packed Produce From Around The Globe for Longevity and Disease Prevention (available in paperback or digital at CIFTofficial.com or Amazon. com) #1 on Amazon in Health and Vitamins category.
- The Energy Healers Oracle—Chapter 3 Intuitive Food Therapy™— Conscious Eating for High Vibrational Wellness #21 of 100 "Best Healing Books of All Time" by Book Authority.

- Feed Your Chakras Vol 1 - 7 (in development).
  Visit CIFTofficial.com for the most updated information.
- Spiritual, Meditation Recording Artist and Producer - Gulf Coast Meditation Series (Available on YouTube & Spotify)
- Gulf Coast Meditations - Awaken the Spirit Within - Track - "Nature"
- Gulf Coast Chaka Meditations - Track - "Third Eye"
- Gulf Coast Abundance Meditations - Track - "Abundance of Healthy Relationships"
- Gulf Coast Meditations Children, Tweens & Teens - Track - "It's All Inside"
- Finn's Giant Leap - Children's Book - Available on Amazon.com

NOURISH YOUR SOUL RETREATS

Join Sevante and guest Healers in exotic locations for retreats around the globe. Retreats are designed to be a sojourn into wellness and a complete rejuvenation of mind, body, and spirit. Cooking classes, food tours, healings, readings, Yoga, meditation, spa, shamanic ceremonies, local excursions await. Visit our FB group and CIFTofficial.com/retreats to learn more.

NOURISH YOUR SOUL AYURVEDA (NYSA)

NYSA is the import brand of pure, organic Ayurvedic teas and incense from Nepal. CIFT – Center for Intuitive Food Therapy™ is the exclusive USA and Canadian importer of Langtang Naturals, a family-owned company's centuries-old formulas for herbal infusions for wellness. Cultivated from herbs grown on farms at the base of the Himalayan mountains, these formulations are now available for the first time in 2024 to buyers in the USA and Canada. To purchase teas and incense, please visit CIFTofficial.com. Selected stores nationwide also carry Nourish Your Soul Teas & Incense.

HOPE FROM THE HIMALAYAS

Sevante is the Executive Producer of this powerful documentary which shares the backstory of the Ayurvedic Teas. *Hope from the Himalayas* focuses on the Nepali Tea Company, Langtang Natural's mission to produce healthy herbal infusions while helping Himalayan Farmers change their belief systems about selling their daughters for trafficking. It's a true story of one man's journey to healing a community steeped in a 200-year-old mindset, one herbal leaf at a time. To learn more and/or make a tax-deductible donation, please visit https://centerforintuitivefoodtherapy.com/himalayas/

NOURISH YOUR SOUL SHOW

Sevante is the host of the Nourish Your Soul Show, an online radio program listened to across the globe now 10 years running. She interviews renowned world healers and spiritual leaders who are moving humanity forward in a positive light. To listen and/or watch, please visit the Nourish Your Soul Show on YouTube or "like" her Nourish Your Soul Show Fb page.

ABOUT THE AUTHOR

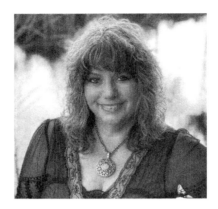

Lainie Sevante Wulkan is Founder of The Center for Intuitive Food Therapy™ (CIFT), Nourish Your Soul Ayurveda & Nourish Your Soul Retreats. She's a multi–modality healer with advanced certifications in Food Healing, Theta Healing and EFT/Tapping. She holds a BS in Food Science, Dietetics & Nutrition from Cal State Northridge and was top of the class in Jeff Primack's "Conquering All Disease Advanced Food Healing" Instructor program. She's an International bestselling Author of *The Food Healing Oracle Deck™* – Nourishing Wisdom from Mother Earth (Co-Authored Vol. 1 & 2) and is writing Volume 3; *Smoothies – Nourishing Wisdom Beyond the Blend, Top Exotic Foods for Natural Healing*. She also wrote a chapter for *The Energy Healers Oracle,* deemed #21 out of 100 best healing books of all time by Book Authority. Sevante is now launching the highly- anticipated seven-volume series, *Feeding Your Chakras* and co-authoring *Angelic Resonance* with International Bestselling Author Angela Orora Medway–Smith.

Sevante elevates humanity by nourishing the mind, body & soul. Her passion is felt throughout all her creations. She offers a deeper knowledge of Spirit and self-expansion to her community to have optimum emotional, mental, physical, and spiritual (EMPS) wellness.

She travels globally with Nourish Your Soul Retreats, speaking at Holistic festivals worldwide, teaching online classes to become a Certified Intuitive Food Therapist, offering private reading and healing sessions, hosting the Nourish Your Soul Show, and expanding her Ayurvedic tea & incense imports from Nepal across USA and Canada.

Sevante is nestled on a beautiful island in Southwest Florida with her husband, Music Producer Howard Merlin Wulkan and their four-legged brood amongst palm trees, enchanted ponds, peacocks and the best of Mother Nature's bounty.

Learn more at www.CIFTofficial.com

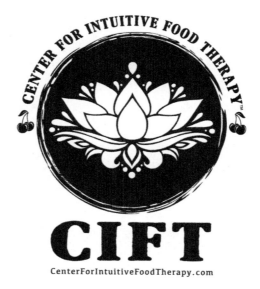

CenterForIntuitiveFoodTherapy.com

*"The true nature of a spiritual being is to recognize enlightened wisdom in our body temple.
When we ignite our powerful intuition and connect with our nourishment needs,
we activate and live life at the highest vibration"*

~ Sevante

Printed in Great Britain
by Amazon

44729975R00159